D0353239

HEALTH VISITING:
TOWARDS COMMUNITY HEALTH NURSING

Withdrawn

Health Visiting: Towards Community Health Nursing

Second Edition

Edited by

KAREN LUKER

BNurs, PhD, RGN, RHV, NDN Cert
Professor of Community Nursing
& Director of the Research and Development Unit
Department of Nursing
University of Liverpool

JEAN ORR

BA, MSc, RGN, RHV, HV Tut Cert
Professor of Nursing
The Queen's University of Belfast
Member of the Health Visiting Joint Committee

OXFORD

BLACKWELL SCIENTIFIC PUBLICATIONS

LONDON EDINBURGH BOSTON

MELBOURNE PARIS BERLIN VIENNA

© 1985, 1992

Blackwell Scientific Publications
Editorial offices:
Osney Mead, Oxford OX2 0EL
25 John Street, London WC1N 2BL
23 Ainslie Place, Edinburgh EH3 6AJ
3 Cambridge Center, Cambridge,
    Massachusetts 02142, USA
54 University Street, Carlton,
    Victoria 3053, Australia

Other Editorial Offices:
Librairie Arnette SA
2, rue Casimir-Delavigne
75006 Paris
France

Blackwell Wissenschafts-Verlag
Meinekestrasse 4
D-1000 Berlin 15
Germany

Blackwell MZV
Feldgasse 13
A-1238 Wien
Austria

All rights reserved. No part of this
publication may be reproduced, stored
in a retrieval system, or transmitted,
in any form or by any means,
electronic, mechanical, photocopying,
recording or otherwise without the
prior permission of the publisher.

First edition published 1985,
reprinted 1986, 1988
This edition published 1992.

Set by DP Photosetting, Aylesbury, Bucks
Printed and bound in Great Britain by
Hartnolls Ltd, Bodmin, Cornwall

DISTRIBUTORS
    Marston Book Services Ltd
    PO Box 87
    Oxford OX2 0DT
    (*Orders:* Tel: 0865 791155
            Fax: 0865 791927
            Telex: 837515)

USA
    Blackwell Scientific Publications, Inc.
    3 Cambridge Center
    Cambridge, MA 02142
    (*Orders:* Tel: 800 759-6102
            617 225-0401)

Canada
    Times Mirror Professional Publishing,
        Ltd
    5240 Finch Avenue East
    Scarborough, Ontario M1S 5A2
    (*Orders:* Tel: 800 268-4178
            416 298-1588)

Australia
    Blackwell Scientific Publications
    (Australia) Pty Ltd
    54 University Street,
    Carlton, Victoria 3053
    (*Orders:* Tel: 03 347-0300)

British Library
Cataloguing in Publication Data
A catalogue record for this book is
available from the British Library.

ISBN 0-632-03324-X

This book is dedicated
to the memory of our Grandmothers

Edith Maud Luker

and

Augustine Davenport

We are privileged to have known them
as outstanding women of their time.

Contents

Foreword

Sarah Andrews, *Director, The Queen's Nursing Institute*

The publication of the second edition of *Health Visiting* coincides with the most significant developments in community nursing this century.

The acknowledgement of community health care nursing as a new entity within the professional discipline of nursing as a whole reflects the changing needs and demands of western society. The practice of community health care nursing, which includes health visiting, district nursing, occupational health nursing and community psychiatric nursing together with a range of additional community nursing specialisms, demands the current educational developments to support it. Proposals outlined in the United Kingdom Central Council's PREPP Reports, combined with changes in practice, are essential dynamic responses to society's changing health needs. These developments will have major and positive effects on health care ensuring the provision of improved services to patients and clients by fully prepared nurses who emphasize the promotion of health and the prevention of ill health as well as therapeutic care for people who are sick or have disability.

The concept of community health care nursing embraces existing and future specialisms relating to the prevailing health needs and demands of national and local population groups, providing for a new and integrated approach to nursing in primary health care. Health visiting is central to the development of the new entity. Firmly placed as part of the family of nursing the underlying principles and skills of health visiting are the essential foundation to effective community health care nursing.

This book demonstrates that community practitioners are vital for the effective provision of primary health care. Working closely with individuals, families and local communities nurses have a significant responsibility to influence health policies and practice. In the complex and ill-defined milieu that is the community, nurses have the local knowledge essential for the appropriate commissioning of health services. They interact with GPs, local authorities and social services, voluntary organisations, the private sector and unpaid carers to ensure a relevant and responsive service provision. They are particularly effective when working with ethnic groups, homeless families and people who are frail, elderly and housebound.

While retaining a health visiting emphasis the editors have introduced new material in this second edition demonstrating that community health care nursing allows for the development of traditional community nursing and health visiting roles. These changes are essential to facilitate flexible working across organizational boundaries and for extending responsibilities in primary care as the NHS and Community Care reforms take effect.

Through group therapy, health centre, clinic, school and workplace intervention as well as home visiting, community practitioners will work actively to promote, conserve, restore and improve people's health. Community practitioners develop and set standards of practice for care of all client populations in all practice settings. They function as clinical specialists and care managers co-ordinating care services within the health care system as a whole, especially at the interface between primary and secondary care. Functioning as teachers, advocates, primary care providers and counsellors, community health care nurses are multi-skilled practitioners who undertake activities resulting in measurable health gains.

This updated text is a timely publication which will be of value for all health visitors and community nurses as they move towards community health care nursing.

May 1992

Introduction

Many changes have occurred in nursing since the publication of the first edition of this book. These changes have been facilitated by the 1979 Nurses and Midwives and Health Visitors Act. A revolution in nursing education has taken place and we now have in place the Project 2000 education programmes. Nurse education now places the emphasis on education and student nurses are students in the true sense of the word. More recently still there have been a number of exciting further developments in terms of links between the traditional colleges of nursing and institutions of further and higher education. in some cases colleges of nursing themselves have moved into higher education, and this can be considered to be a major step forward for the development of nursing as a profession.

Interestingly, one of the major shifts in the Project 2000 curriculum is an emphasis on health and community. Diplomates from these courses are expected to be able to function at a first level both in hospital and the community   again an exciting development. While many nurses may not currently be engaged in community assessment, health promotion and anticipatory care, there is a new emphasis in basic nurse education and this gives 'community health' a prominence which previously it has not received. These changes can be expected to ultimately reshape the education and practice of all nurses, health visitors and midwives working in the community.

Now that Project 2000 is being implemented the focus has turned to post-registration education and practice and the UK Central Council (UKCC) is leading on the proposals set out in the Post Registration Education and Practice Project (PREPP, UKCC 1990) report. As part of this it was agreed to form a subgroup of PREPP looking at community education and practice.

It is important to set the scene in which the subgroup carried out its task. There is an increasing concern about the future role of community nurses as a result of the NHS and Community Care Act 1990 and the Children Act 1989. The introduction of a market economy in health care has made people question both the value of community nursing services

1

and whether there might be cheaper options available. It is difficult to fit a public health dimension within a market model of health care.

As a result of the new GP contract there is a rise in the number of practice nurses; at the same time, secondment to all community nursing courses is falling. The increasing move towards skill mix in the community has caused concern about the ratio of trained to untrained staff and what this will mean for client care.

Since Project 2000 nurses are prepared to work in either hospitals or the community, there was a fear that there may not be a need for additional education beyond initial registration. It was against this background that the PREPP subgroup produced their report (UKCC 1991).

Firstly, the subgroup decided that the title given to all nurses working in the community should be 'community health care nurse'. This is intended as an overall title to describe the setting in which the care is given – in much the same way that nurses in ward situations are called hospital nurses. It is envisaged that existing health visitors will keep their name. It is important that they do so because the power of naming in society is such that it shapes the reality and places workers in a historical context.

Secondly, there is a need to have a range of nurses to meet the health care needs of the future. There is no doubt that many health visitors have been worried about the idea that there should be one generic title 'community nurse', particularly as the implication is that this nurse would not be solely involved in health promotion.

The report makes clear that the complexity of the work to be undertaken in the community requires nurses who have specialist skills and knowledge. It was felt impossible that one nurse should be able to deliver high quality care across a range of clients and situations.

Thirdly, the report states that a Project 2000 nurse should be able to work as a first-level nurse under the direction of the qualified community nurse. This reaffirms the fact that there will need to be a system of further education in order to qualify nurses to work in different specialities within the community.

Fourthly, there will be a range of routes to such preparation, depending on the background and experience of the students. For example, at present we only take students from the general register but now we will be able to select from all four branches as well as from midwifery. The main framework will be that of a range of modules forming a common core; from this students will be able to exercise some choice depending on their previous experience. A number of modules, such as health visiting/health promotion, will then make up the specialist element of the preparation.

To summarize, the key features of the proposals set out in the report are as follows:

- New unified discipline of community health care nursing.
- New shared common core (across the range of practice) with specialist modules to prepare for discrete areas of practice.
- Greater flexibility and choice for practitioners and employers.
- Increased opportunities for enrolled nurses.
- Recognition of existing community practitioners.

The advantages are seen as follows:

- Matching clinical responsibility with tailored preparation which will improve standards of care for patients, clients and their families.
- Recording a qualification in community health care nursing on the UKCC Register which will both protect standards and indicate skill.
- Creating a rational and cost-effective framework which makes more efficient, effective and economic use of resources and which embraces the range of post-registration nursing education and practice.
- Providing a more flexible and more sensitive means of ensuring that education is relevant and responsive to health and service need.

Because of these proposed changes, at present going through the consultation process, the title of this book has been broadened even further to take account of the recommendations; health visiting is thus seen as one element of community health care nursing.

In addition to the revolution in nursing education, community nursing is greatly affected by the National Health Service and Community Care Act (1990). At the time of preparing this second edition we have not had the opportunity to fully experience all the implications. The renewed emphasis on effectiveness and efficiency, and on quality control, has led to the emergence of different models of health care: some hospitals and community units, for example, have opted for NHS trust status, and we await with interest the outcome of these initiatives. General managers are now in the position of firming up contracts to provide pre-specified services to a variety of purchasers. We are optimistic that, in the end, consumers will receive a better quality of service as a result of these efforts.

The District Health Authorities are charged with securing measurable improvements in the health of their resident population. There are a number of important factors which District Health Authorities must take into account as they determine local priorities. The separate but linked elements in these assessments are:

(1)   Epidemiological assessments based on the ability to benefit from health care and which reflect what is known about incidence, prevalence and the effectiveness of treatment including cost effectiveness.
(2)   Comparative assessments by which District Health Authorities look at performance, price and utilization to indicate the need for change. This category would include the use of demographic data.
(3)   There is now a 'corporate' view which takes account of the interests of local people, GPs, providers and their clinical staff, other agencies such as the FHSA (Family Health Services Authority), Regions and the NHS Management Executive.

Drawing on these elements, District Health Authorities will be able to make an overall assessment of the health of the local population and establish local priorities. Their service specifications can then outline proposals for change as the basis for contracting. Because it will take some time to develop epidemiological assessments, District Health Authorities are being encouraged to develop a systematic approach by using indicators which already exist, by comparing performance within and across districts, and by developing contacts with other agencies which will help to produce a corporate local view of priorities. It is seen to be important that there are good working arrangements with FHSAs because the responsibilities of the two authorities are closely linked: examples of this are most likely to be in the field of health promotion. In a recent District Health Authority Project Paper produced by the NHS Management Executive (NHS 1991) the following six questions set out what the District Health Authorities need to answer:

(1)   What do we know about the health problems and services in the district?
(2)   What issues and changes in service should we focus on?
(3)   What do we want to achieve?
(4)   How can we make it happen?
(5)   What have we agreed with our providers?
(6)   What is happening under our contracts?

It would seem to be important for health visitors to feed into the needs assessment by looking at incidence and prevalence of particular conditions within the community and making the voices of the local population heard. The Project Paper states that developing links with local people will be essential as District Health Authorities take forward their new role. Thus they will need to develop the means to:

(1) Discover and respond to the views of local people about the pattern and delivery of services, distinguishing between users' views and general public opinion.
(2) Describe and explain the District Health Authorities' objectives as they take forward service changes.

The providers of services will have their own views on the initiatives they want to include in their own business plans. They will also be able to give their own perceptions of purchaser priorities compared to the day-to-day demands placed on their services. It is therefore important that the opinions of clinical staff are heard.

It is interesting that within the document there is no specific reference to community nursing, although the report does state that District Health Authorities will neither have the resources of staff nor the skills to carry out the work necessary to lead informed change. It will be necessary for them therefore to have a co-operative relationship between not only the Health Authorities but also with Social Services Departments. The choice of areas for priority attention will be made on the basis of an overall assessment of the local situation using the three elements of needs assessment – epidemiology, comparative and corporate. This may include some service priority because of its historical or political importance. We should be in no doubt, however, that existing services cannot be guaranteed. The directors of public health have a statutory responsibility to produce an annual report on the health of the local population which picks out key issues. The choice of areas as priorities for fundamental review will not imply that they will receive extra resources. District Health Authorities may choose areas for attention where they believe better value for money might be obtained or services might be better structured. This emphasis on cost effectiveness and value for money poses a dilemma for health visiting.

The community care proposals also have implications for health visitors as they will have a major role in assessing need and managing care in co-operation with Social Services. In this context, need is seen as 'the requirement of individuals to enable them to achieve, maintain or restore an acceptable level of social independence or quality of life as defined by the particular care agency or authority' (DOH 1991). Within this document it states that a considerable amount of negotiation may be required to develop collaborative care management and assessment procedures. The Government has not thought it appropriate to attempt to define rigid demarcation between health and social care and the interface between the two will be a matter for local discussion and agreement.

The section on community nursing states that there will be even greater demands on the community nursing services if the objective of maintaining more dependent people in the community for longer periods is to be achieved. This is said to be likely to reinforce the trend towards nurses working in teams with a broad skill mix that more closely mirrors social services social work teams. The guide states that community nurses, as well as assessing nursing care needs, may also act as care managers.

The section on training states that it is vital that each agency does not develop a training strategy in isolation from that of other agencies but that at every stage opportunities are taken to identify common training needs and shared means of addressing them. 'Joint training', it is further stated, will become one of the most effective ways of ensuring a more collaborative approach to community care.

Perhaps the most significant change in the 1990s to impact on the work of health visitors has been the new contract issued to general practitioners. This contract places GPs at the centre of primary health care rather than primary medical care and the newly formed Family Health Service Authorities (FHSA) are charged with wider responsibilities than the old Family Practitioner Committees (FPC). Consequent upon these changes there has been an escalation of the numbers of practice nurses employed. The numbers are such that it has led many other community nurses to reflect on their own contribution to care and in some cases there has been a re-negotiation of role boundaries.

GPs are charged with the responsibility of ensuring that patients registered with their practice have access to preventive health care. Unfortunately, some health visitors have found these developments threatening. It would seem that one of the major challenges facing health professionals in the community is to learn to work together in a more effective manner and this will inevitably involve transcending traditional professional boundaries. Furthermore, the success of the reforms embodied in the new NHS and Community Care Act will depend on intersectorial collaboration; this is perhaps best illustrated by thinking of the potential overlap between nursing and social services in the provision of care to the frail and elderly living at home.

Although many individual nurses are still quite anxious about the future, the general feeling seems to be that there is more than enough work for everyone. In some areas, for example, practice nurses have agreed to joint protocols for visiting the elderly for screening and health promotion as well as systems for keeping each other informed about exactly who is doing what.

The attitude of district health authority community nursing services towards the new contract seems to determine how well or badly staff collaborate on the ground. Initially, there was talk of charging GPs for the services of their attached health visitors and district nurses since the new contract coincided with community units having to quantify and cost their services and draw up business plans.

This idea now seems to have given way to a desire to make community nurses available (if not indispensable) to GPs. Many District Health Authorities are entering into service agreements with practices as to what input community staff will make, thus reviving the Cumberlege (1986) proposal (not at all welcomed by GPs at the time it was first made). Most District Health Authorities have sought to maintain the status quo as far as attachment is concerned; many of them do not have sufficient resources to provide attached staff where practices had not previously wanted them.

There are no hard data yet to indicate what impact the contract is having on the work of the majority of health visitors and district nurses; nor is there evidence to suggest any significant change in their professional roles. Even if there were, this would be difficult to judge because of the confounding effects of all the other changes currently taking place in relation both to the structure and organization of community health services and to developments in professional practice.

The need, for example, for District Health Authorities to clear financial deficits has led to reductions in some areas of child clinic sessions, fewer sessions with a clinical medical officer in attendance, and vacant health visitor caseloads. So if more mothers take their children to the GP for immunization and check-ups, is this because they want to or because they have no alternative? In other areas, the development of more user-friendly services is increasing District Health Authority clinic attendance, in spite of the extreme pressure which some GPs are reported to be exerting on patients to go to them for these services.

The structure of community nursing services

Over the past few years there has been an ongoing debate on the best way of organizing the range of community nursing services to meet the needs of the population. There are two reports which are central to this debate, the Cumberlege Report and the Roy Report.

The Cumberlege Report (1986) was one of the most important

documents on community nursing to be published in the last ten years and it is sad that it has not been implemented more fully. The imperative of the report required that nursing start by defining client and community needs and deciding among teams of nurses how these needs could be met. This involved setting priorities and deciding which nurses or team had the appropriate skills. The concept challenged us to work in a collective way with a range of nurses and emphasized the primacy of nursing in its widest sense rather than that of medicine. Because of its significance, it is important to look at some aspects of the report in detail as well as at its list of recommendations.

The Cumberlege Report stressed that the primary health care services should enable people to make decisions about their health on the basis of informed choice, and should also involve partnership with and support for carers and all disciplines and statutory and voluntary services, as well as to ensure that the planning and evaluation of services involves people in the community as well as health professionals.

Cumberlege suggested that community nursing be centred on geographical areas that were spatially determined by natural community boundaries. These neighbourhoods, with populations of 10 000 to 25 000, would be served by neighbourhood nursing teams incorporating district nurses, school nurses and health visitors. In this way, existing lines of demarcation would be broken down so that, for example, district nurses could supervise preventive screening programmes for older people. This new approach would be facilitated by providing common core education for community nurses.

The report highlights the criticism, particularly by health visitors, of the outcome of general practice attachment. While Cumberlege stated that primary health care teams and general practice attachment were ideally the best way to deliver care, it recognized that properly functioning teams are few and far between. It also recognized that many health visitors were moving to a more community-centred approach not just because of dissatisfaction with the illness-orientation of GP attachment, but because it is recognized that what affects health is located in the community and that the resources of the community networks are a vital part of care. It can also be easier to identify at-risk groups within the community and to provide group facilities for delivering health promotion. The Report further states that:

'We see district nurses, health visitors and school nurses, with their support staff, working together as an integrated nursing team. Individually, they would still work closely with general practitioners, but, as part also of a nursing team, they could, we believe, become a major force for change and improvement in community health services.

Apart from other benefits, which we will describe, the neighbourhood nursing service would bring school nursing in from the periphery of primary care; it would mean that the needs of a neighbourhood's children would be brought into much sharper focus and would make it easier to take a more integrated, family-based approach to the health care of children and young people.

Having identified particular health needs in the community, the members of the neighbourhood nursing services would be able to bring relevant problems and ideas for solutions to their general practitioner colleagues for individual or joint action. At the same time, general practitioners would have access to more nursing skills than are normally available in a smaller primary health care team working alone.'

The recommendations (listed in Appendix 5) have not been implemented in full. The major opposition to the report came from GPs who objected strongly to the suggestion that subsidies should no longer be paid to them to employ staff to perform nursing duties. As it has turned out, as a result of the GP contract, the increase in practice nurses is causing concern because there are few safeguards to protect the public from nurses who may be working beyond the limit of their competence in what is a professionally isolated situation.

It is impossible to say at this time what the future shape of health services in general and community services in particular will be after the introduction of the NHS and Community Care Act 1990. However, it is likely to be very different to that which we already know. The major influences are the GP contract, the increase in the number of practice nurses, the changing role of Family Health Services Authorities (FHSA) and the workings of the internal market in health and social care. The irony for nurses is that there was very little mention of nursing, midwifery or health visiting in the White Papers (DOH 1989b and 1989c), and yet these services may be radically changed with very little debate with either the professionals or the clients. It is in response to this concern that the Roy Report was produced in 1990.

'The Report, initiated by Health Minister Virginia Bottomley, covers the management of district nurses, health visitors, community midwives, CPNs, community mental handicap nurses, school nurses and other community specialists. It also includes GP-based practice nurses across the range of organisation structures within which they work.

The five models suggested are:

1   *The Stand Alone Community Trust or Directly Managed Unit (DMU)* – a community unit to manage all community health services and offer them to GPs, secondary care units, local authority, voluntary agencies and the independent sector on a contractual basis.

2   *Locality Management/Neighbourhood Nursing model* – mixed teams of community staff managed in geographical patches or around consortia of GP practices; under the overall control of a trust/DMU, or managed separately. GPs would continue to employ practice nurses in a complementary way.

3   *Expanded FHSA model* – FHSA to assume responsibility for provision of community services under an agency arrangement with the DHA. GPs would employ practice nurses and tap into more specialised community services for forms of care the practice nurse did not provide. In exceptional circumstances, the FHSA might directly employ staff.

4   *Vertical Integration or Outreach Model* – could be in various combinations of acute/community unit, with either community or acute unit as outreach. Current examples include mental health/ mental illness units and elderly care units. Here purchasing authorities would contract with DMUs or trusts to provide complete packages of care, including discharge management.

5   *Primary Health Care Team (PHCT)* – GP-managed community services to be brought under control and management of general practice. Model could be centred around individual practices, consortia of GPs or health centre.' (Roy 1990)

The report sets out a number of differing options and is fair in its consideration of the pros and cons of each model. The report quite clearly stresses the importance of management, and must be encouraging to those nursing managers who have felt themselves under threat.

Whichever option is decided upon it is clear that the world of community nursing will never be the same again. The key management principles which are said to underpin a good service are a shared vision of care; commitment to joint working and putting patients first; joint assessments of population needs; joint strategies; effective communications and commitment to quality.

Can these be achieved in a market system which is about competition? In considering the models there are a number of questions to be asked.

Do all models expect the same outcomes in terms of client care? If they do, we need to know the imperatives determining the choice of a model. Will the choice be based on professional power? For example, the GP-managed model clearly has implications for community nursing. On the positive side we may welcome the idea of joining GPs as equal partners but would be less happy with the prospect of being employed by GPs. The vertical integration or outreach model – also known as clinical directorates – would threaten the focus of work with the well population and could let the acute sector dominate the service. This model could pose problems in fragmenting the services and make it difficult to work at a community level. The model which appears to be gaining favour is the expanded FHSA one. Some FHSAs are already employing nurse managers to take developments forward and manage the growing number of practice nurses.

New movements in public health

There are a number of major movements gaining popularity in the public health field which broaden the health debate and challenge some of our accepted ways of looking at the issues. One of the early proponents of what has been called health public policy has been Nancy Milio (1986) who addressed the issues of environment, energy, ecology and agriculture policy as they affected health. Milio, a Professor of Nursing in America, has influenced the World Health Organisation (WHO) thinking on health promotion policy. She saw health policy as public policy that affects health and not just health services. Milio states:

> 'Policy is after all no more nor no less than a collective choice on collective lifestyle that sets the terms for individual choices ... public policy has been and is now more than ever affecting profiles of health and illness, who shall be healthy and how healthy'.

Hancock and Duhl (1985) see a public policy on health as questioning the 'givens' in society such as how do we have to structure our society so as to create health? These are very challenging questions and point up the inequalities in society which not all political parties wish to acknowledge.

The Public Health Alliance (Blane, 1989), a national movement to bring together individuals and organizations to promote and redefine public health in the United Kingdom, was launched in 1987. It has produced a Charter identifying ten principles which are seen as the rights of every citizen as a means to maintain good health:

(1) An income which provides the material means to maintain health.
(2) Homes that are safe, warm and dry.
(3) Food that is safe, nourishing, widely available and cheap.
(4) Transport that permits accessible safe travel at a reasonable cost.
(5) Work that is properly rewarded in or out of the home and free from hazards to health and safety.
(6) Environments protected from dangerous pollution and radiation and planned to preserve and enhance our quality of life.
(7) Public services which provide for those who need it.
(8) Education and health promotion.
(9) Comprehensive health services properly resourced.
(10) Equal opportunities to good health regardless of class, race, sex, physical ability, age or sexual orientation.

The above points are all important ones that community nurses must take into account in their work with families and communities.

There is an important movement known informally as 'the new public health' which has implications for community nurses. Draper (1991), in setting out the key issues for health through public policy, shows the links between health and economics, trade, politics, international relations, agriculture, transport, energy, planning and freedom of information.

Draper outlines six general characteristics of this new public health:

(1) Several sectors are often involved in a given health area and therefore health has a multisectional focus.
(2) Health policy needs to involve commerce and industry, voluntary organizations and the general public as well as central and local government.
(3) Health hazards are not confined within national and regional boundaries.
(4) The aim of health policy is to be educational and persuasive rather than dictatorial or puritanical.
(5) Community health initiatives are an important part of health policy.
(6) Health public policy is intrinsically political but not party political.

The 'Healthy Cities' project

The 'Healthy Cities' project has been described by Ashton and Seymour (1985) as:

'a new European WHO initiative which is intended to lend support to city-based health promotion. The project has its origins in the World Health Organization Strategy of *Health For All by the Year 2000* and is based on the 38 European targets for health for all. The European project is a collaborative one between the health promotion and environmental health sections of WHO. It has a particular emphasis on the promotion of healthy environments and lifestyles. The role of WHO in the project will be to act as a catalyst and facilitator in the process of agenda-setting, consciousness-raising and establishing models of good practice'.

The 'Healthy Cities' project contains five major elements:

(1) The formulation of concepts leading to the adoption of city plans for health which are action-based and which use *Health For All*, health promotion principles and the 38 European targets as a framework.
(2) The development of models of good practice which represent a variety of different entry points in action depending on cities' own perceived priorities. These may range from major environmental action to programmes designed to support individual lifestyle change, but they illustrate the key principles of health promotion.
(3) Monitoring and research into the effectiveness of models of good practice on health in cities.
(4) Dissemination of ideas and experiences between collaborating cities and other interested cities.
(5) Mutual support, collaboration and learning, and cultural exchange between the towns and cities of Europe (Ashton *et al.*, 1986).

Labonte (1986) argues that health is primarily an outcome of socio-economic structures and that public health must become a moral voice in the struggle to end social inequality. Within this framework, health education is explicitly political and based primarily on working with community groups to bring about social change. Labonte sees the implication of such an agreement as meaning that the health educator should be a 'community agitator' who not only works with the health groups but with groups such as feminists, trade unionists, and minority rights groups. The health educator should also be as critically analytical as possible in charting out the health implications of policy and change. Thirdly, health educators must be conversant with the politics, science and policies of toxic substances and must use multiple strategies in reducing public health risks.

This radical approach to health education poses challenges to health care workers but indicates the way we must be thinking in order to affect change in the nation's health (Moran, 1991). Moran sees the GP contract's focus on payment for meeting health targets as an example of a simplistic market mechanism which is not appropriate and which takes a narrow vision of the public health potential of primary care reducing it to a series of technical medical interventions which ignores the wider social and economic conditions which affect people's lives. As Moran points out, there are no bonus payments for GPs who highlight poor housing, poverty or unemployment. Some districts may develop imaginative initiatives in collaboration with other agencies but this will take considerable input from those professionals who value public health.

The developments within the 'Healthy Cities' initiatives and the new public health are central to the future of health visiting. The 'Health of the Nation' (DOH 1991a), a discussion paper produced by the Government, demonstrates an interest in and focus on prevention and targeting and has set the agenda for health care in the future. Key health areas identified include:

- Coronary heart disease
- Stroke
- Cancers
- Smoking
- Eating and drinking
- Prevention of accidents
- Pregnant women and children
- Diabetes
- Mental health
- Rehabilitation
- Asthma

This is the type of initiative that fits into the work and expertise of health visitors or indeed community health nurses. In many respects, the changes which have occurred in the structure and provision of community health care have highlighted the importance of the skills and knowledge of the health visitor, in so far as the principles of health visiting practice have in part been assimilated into other branches of community health nursing. It has taken many years, but now it seems that the issues which surround the provision of preventive health care in the community have been recognized as important by hospital nurses and others. Health promotion and community assessment will now form part of basic nursing education.

The first edition of this book was well received and was reprinted three times. The feedback which we have received suggested that the book was rather futuristic. It is interesting that in the intervening six years many of the issues we raised are now current topics. The most notable examples are community level assessment and the issues surrounding outcome evaluation. It is interesting also to note that the so-called 'new public health' (Ashton & Seymour, 1988) strongly emphasizes the importance of community health assessments and community participation. Our observation has been that most health visitors do not as yet engage in this level of practice; local policy prefers to give pre-eminence to the individual or family rather than the group. However, with the appointment of the first public health nurse in Liverpool in 1990, we see an increasing need for health visitors to update their skills on community health assessment. In the light of current health policy, Chapter 5, on the subject of evaluation, will probably make a more important contribution in the 1990s than it did in the 1980s.

A major addition to this text is the chapter on information technology in relation to community health nursing. The collection of information is already a central aspect of community nursing work and all nurses will find that information technology (IT) will become increasingly important in their work. Hence, no book which seeks to deal with issues in health visiting should go to press without coverage of this topic.

There is a fundamental shift in basic nurse education which will have far-reaching implications for health visiting practice and education. The period of the next five years promises to be an extremely exciting time in health visiting.

Karen Luker
Jean Orr

1   Knowledge and Practice of Working in the Community

Kathleen Robinson, PhD, BA, SRN, HV, *Dean of Health Care and Social Studies, Luton College of Higher Education*

THE NATURE OF KNOWLEDGE

Where does nursing knowledge come from? Is nursing knowledge generated through scientific activity? Is there a theory of nursing, and what aspect of nursing knowledge is unique? These are important questions which nurses are beginning to take seriously. Although nurses are primarily people who act, we know that action without thought is likely to be, at best, inefficient and, at worst, dangerous. So it is important that we understand from the start what the concept of knowledge means. Knowledge is not an object that is acquired and possessed like a tin of beans or a packet of biscuits. We cannot 'buy' knowledge and just put it away in some store cupboard in the mind ready for the planned lunch or unexpected tea party. Our knowledge is not a simple reflection of the 'reality' of the world. The world has no intrinsic meaning and order until we construct such meanings and create order.

Knowledge is often referred to as perspective, framework, philosophy or ideology. For example, we talk of: a sociological perspective of the family, ideology of the Welfare State, a nursing process framework. However, the choice of the term we use is essentially arbitrary.

Knowledge can be defined as the process of knowing or the process of organizing our experience. It is a dynamic activity rather than a static entity. This dynamic characteristic of knowledge is illustrated by the anecdote in which the famous philosopher Popper instructed his class to 'observe'. The students found the apparently simple task impossible to perform – 'observe what?' they asked (Magee, 1973). Similarly, student community nurses may share the bewilderment of Popper's class when asked to assess family needs. Assess what? they may well ask. It is impossible to define facts and events without a framework, i.e. a knowledge base which defines and categorizes objects and occurrences, experiences and feelings, in a meaningful way. This framework includes all the theories, organizing principles and philosophies which structure our experience. It incorporates both knowing how and knowing that

(Ryle, 1963). Only from inside such a framework can we see certain events as important and others as trivial, or define individual events as being characteristic of a set of activities. The framework allows us to define, label, categorize and codify all our experiences, whether they are of the natural or the social world. It is a 'map' which organizes our activities and progress, although we must remember that this 'map' is in practice always changing unless frozen in time by, for example, being produced as a book or given as a lecture.

As the knowledge framework we use assigns meaning to the external world, then obviously we cannot appeal to that external 'reality' in order to assess the truth or falsity of our descriptions of it. Like meaning, truth is socially constructed and socially evaluated. Medical diagnoses, for example, are not simple readings of the labels of the biological world. They are products of social thinking and negotiation about what we want to label and how and why (Wright & Treacher, 1982). Thus medical labels change both over time and between cultures.

As nurses we are familiar with controversial medical diagnoses such as alcoholism and homosexuality, and with diagnoses that are no longer in current use. Figlio (1982), for example, has documented the use of the medical diagnosis of 'miner's nystagmus' which is unknown today but in the 1920s and 1930s 'had become the most expensive item of compensation in the mining industry, and the Medical Research Council prepared three reports on it.' The important point which Figlio illustrates is that any medical diagnosis is a social process and therefore potentially open to reassessment and redefinition. Myalgic encephalitis (ME) gives us a recent example of a disease category which is still being negotiated. No one doubts that there are individuals who feel ill and have a range of symptoms which they dislike: the question is whether we construct it as an illness or simply as 'the sort of thing which happens to people from time to time' its final status in the medical system remains in doubt.

So knowledge exists only as an active constituent of human life; as a means by which we cope with and define and indeed construct the social reality which surrounds us. It is like a house in which we live and from which we look out at the world. At any one time the windows of the house allow us to see only certain vistas, but because we can redesign and rebuild the house we have potential access to great variety and change in our surroundings. It is because the reconstruction of our knowledge framework is such an active process that completing the health visiting, or a community nursing course, may be such a demanding and difficult endeavour.

The various facets of the complex concept of knowledge has been usefully summarized by Shibutani (1955) as:

An ordered view of one's world - what is taken for granted about the attributes of various objects, events and human nature. It is an order of things remembered and expected as well as things actually perceived, an organised conception of what is plausible and what is possible; it constitutes the matrix through which one perceives his environment.

SCIENCE VERSUS COMMONSENSE KNOWLEDGE

The distinction between science, and social or commonsense knowledge has become institutionalized. Science or academic knowledge has acquired privileged status which is maintained through institutions like universities and medical schools. The special status of science is enhanced and legitimized by the scientists' claim that scientific knowledge is better, that is, more true, than the commonsense knowledge we use in our everyday lives. The commonsense observation that the earth remains still while the sun moves, for instance, is refuted by the scientific observation that the earth revolves around the sun, and indeed both are hurtling through space at enormous speeds. The claim to superiority is based on the notion that scientists are 'objective', that they 'stand outside' the commonsense world and, using strict rules of procedure and logic known as the scientific method, produce 'real' descriptions of either the natural or the social world. Commonsense knowledge, on the other hand, has less strict rules of procedure and is concerned less with the complete understanding of any phenomenon than with having enough knowledge to 'get by' or to make things work. When you ask a lay person, for instance, how the spindryer works you are more likely to be told which knob to press rather than be given a lecture of centrifugal force.

It is important to be clear about the extent of the differences between science and commonsense knowledge and about the relevance of the differences. In general, it is becoming clear that the claims of scientists may have been overestimated. For instance, the emphasis on objectivity overestimates the extent to which commonsense knowledge can be excluded from the activity of scientists. Scientists are still people living in the social world and they must use as many of the concepts and theories of the ordinary world to operate even as scientists (Elliot, 1974). Similarly, it is not true to say that only scientists theorize and construct models. Commonsense knowledge is also the product of original commonsense theorizing. Although it is true that generally we conduct our affairs according to 'recipes' for action (Schutz, 1964) which allow us to act in a relatively unselfconscious and automatic fashion, recipes originally arose from commonsense theorizing. When we meet unfamiliar phenomena or need to act in unfamiliar surroundings where there is no 'recipe' available for use, we can all start to theorize and construct models and hypotheses to account for unfamiliar phenomena. Scientists tend to do this more selfconsciously and more frequently, but it is not a uniquely scientific skill. Most importantly, any claim that one particular form of knowledge is 'better than' another should provoke the question 'better for what purpose?' The apparently disinterested pursuit of pure knowledge has certainly been very valuable in some areas of life, but often events will not wait for such a lengthy process of investigation. In any case, scientific investigation is concerned with events in general rather than any particular case or instance. Instant action through commonsense recipes or theories is therefore both necessary and usually adequate. Many situations can be managed without perfect understanding. Magellan circumnavigated the globe before Newtonian cosmology explained how it was possible. Similarly the mother with a crying infant is not interested in a scientific explanation of why babies in general cry, she merely wants to help *her* baby.

Group knowledge

An individual does not have to create an entirely original perspective on the world by building new categories and distinctions to make sense of the environment. Each individual is born into membership of an existing social group possessing a distinct body of knowledge. This provides a pre-existing scheme for interpreting the world and guidelines for suitable ways of acting in it. The distinction between individual and group knowledge is therefore made to simplify analysis. They are each facets of the same knowledge framework: an individual's knowledge must be part of a group's knowledge, and any group consists of a number of individuals.

A social framework of knowledge is not merely a set of rules dictating behaviour. Rather it is a potentially flexible and negotiable system of guidelines which are subject to change. However, within the group, control over knowledge will be differentially distributed. Some members will be given particular power over defining and passing on the knowledge, or particular sections of it, while others are excluded from any influence or choice. In this context nurses may be considered privileged since they are assumed by society to have particular expertise which they may choose to pass on to particular chosen groups, i.e. their students, or in selective ways to their clients. The consumer movement can be seen in part as a challenge to this idea that groups can keep their knowledge to themselves. Attempts by the excluded segments to change either their own or the group's perspective may be met with sanctions such as incarceration in prison or mental hospitals or compulsory re-education. This question of differential power will be discussed later on in this chapter.   \

However, the pressure for change in group knowledge is not as great as the word 'negotiate' might imply because the framework for interpreting the world appears to the members inside the group to be a stable and inevitable account of reality. It has the appearance of an accurate representation of the way things really are. Each group framework viewed from inside appears normal and rational, but from outside it may seem ridiculous and irrational.

Schutz (1964) in his essay 'The Stranger' comments that:

'Any member born or reared within the group accepts the ready-made standards and schema of the cultural pattern handed down to him by ancestors, teachers, and authorities as an unquestioned and unques-tionable guide in all situations which normally occur within the social world.'

Schutz goes on to describe the difficulties of the transition from one taken-for-granted system of knowledge to another. He takes as his example the position of the immigrant, i.e., the stranger in a new land. The immigrant very soon discovers that things in the new surroundings look quite different from what they were expected to be. This is frequently the first shock to the immigrant's confidence. His usual thinking pattern, that is the framework he habitually uses to make sense of the world, has to be revised if he is to survive in the new land (Schutz, 1964).

Students might gain insight into their own position by reading this essay. It can be argued that neophyte community health nursing students are indeed strangers to the world of community nursing and newcomers to the world of higher education. Students very soon come to realize that their previous nursing experience may in fact hinder, rather than help, their passage into the community.

Our society contains many specialized bodies of knowledge and therefore the strangeness of transition between systems of knowledge described by Schutz is a common experience. Such bodies of group knowledge may relate to particular occupations, such as teaching or law, or they may relate to particular methods of producing validating and transmitting the knowledge, as in religion or science. It is interesting to note that the ability of one person to move readily between separate bodies of knowledge is a relatively recent phenomenon. For instance, the Japanese samurai was born into his role and defined himself as a samurai at all times; and it would be impossible for him to lay down his swords and become a fisherman even for one day. However, in our society the scientist who acts in her everyday world as she does in the laboratory is an accepted vehicle for caricature. For in our society it is expected that we play several different roles and use different knowledge. A woman, for example, may have several roles, a manager at work, while at home she is a mother and wife and to the nurse she is a client.

Occupational knowledge

Occupational knowledge is a form of group knowledge that is 'owned' by an occupational group (Sharrock, 1974). It provides the framework by which the occupational members define their goals and activities. It provides a number of theories and recipes for action. There are variations in the degree to which any occupation is allowed to monopolize any particular area of knowledge and to legally enforce this monopoly. In general, the more secure the monopoly, as in scientific medicine, the more 'professional' the group is deemed to be. However, exclusive knowledge, like any other form of property, is a scarce resource and society will express and reinforce existing relationships of power and control through the distribution of knowledge.

An occupational body of knowledge is not a scientific body of knowledge, for it contains notions of occupational priorities and goals which are not compatible with any scientific notion of detachment or with the scientific goal of complete understanding. Occupations exist to organize activity, and understanding is a secondary priority pursued in order to aid more efficient or efficacious action. The assertion that such knowledge is not scientific is not synonymous with saying that it is irrational or immature or 'wrong'. The claim is simply that it is different, since it uses different methods to pursue different goals.

Sources of occupational knowledge

Where does the knowledge of any occupational group come from? This will vary depending on the nature of the occupation, but there are three main sources, as follows:

(1) There are the everyday theories current in ordinary life. For example, there are theories about the nature of motherhood and what counts as competent mothering.

(2)   There are theories derived from basic scientific disciplines such as psychology and physiology. Obvious examples include theories of human development, and the germ theory of disease.
(3)   There are the occupational theories produced by practitioners which are generated in response to experiences of practice, and may be taken up and preserved by the whole group. For example, theories about what constitutes an adequate home visit.

This is a greatly simplified description of a complex situation, and perhaps suggests too strongly that the occupations can draw freely from a variety of sources. It needs to be realized that no occupation exists in a social vacuum. Each occupation is sustained and supported by the social environment of which it is a part. And it is involved with negotiating its role, purpose and power in that wider social context. Its freedom of action may also be severely constrained by the prior existence of another ideology already operating in its particular field. This may be the situation in which nursing finds itself in relation to the power of medical knowledge.

The exact routes by which scientific ideas come to be accepted as commonsense, or are accepted into specialized areas of professional competence, are different in every case. Occupations may establish direct links with the producers of scientific findings, for instance, by providing publishing facilities in occupational journals. Alternatively, organizations may mediate between them. The drug companies, for instance, mediate between research chemists and doctors, and the DOH mediates between scientists and health care workers in the production of guidelines for practice.

The relationship between scientific, everyday and occupational knowledge has been discussed by Berger (1965) in his interesting essay 'Towards a Sociological Understanding of Psychoanalysis'. Berger discusses how the original ideas of psychoanalysis propounded by Freud have come to permeate many layers of cultural thought. He suggests that psychoanalytic concepts such as 'the unconscious', 'repression', 'frustration', and 'needs' have become taken for granted as 'real' entities whose existence is unquestionable. He also cites the germ theory of disease as an example of a similar scientific theory which has become accepted into society as a description of reality. Although Berger is talking about events in the United States his account is equally relevant here.

The articulation of occupational knowledge

An occupational body of knowledge has an existence apart from the individual actions of the occupational members. Through being pre-served in oral and written traditions, and especially by being organized as a syllabus or instructional framework for new members, it comes to have a certain stability and permanence. It may be called an occupational philosophy or ideology. Despite this apparent stability any occupational knowledge remains knowledge-in-use, and it will be presented and articulated differently on each occasion of its use, depending on the nature and purpose of the occasion. Each presentation of a community health nursing perspective will therefore be unique and yet must also remain recognizably and legitimately inside a community health nursing framework. It will be an individual interpretation of a unique occasion and yet part of a strong cognitive tradition. Health visiting knowledge, for example, will be manifested in professional statements about the nature of health visiting. It will be presented to students during training. It will form the basis of talk between practicing health visitors in any clinic; it will be interwoven into any talk between health visitor and client; and it will form the basis of management judgments and decisions. The same goes for practice nurses and other community nurses.

None of these presentations however, is the correct or complete one. A description of an occupational knowledge base will always be a compo-site one, composed of analyses of many different occasions of use. Such a description would probably find variations in the occupational

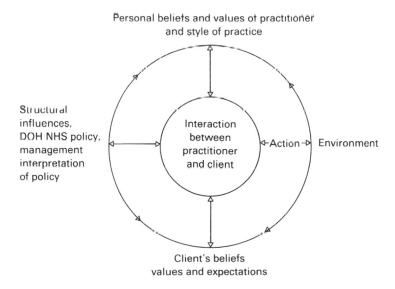

Fig. 1.1. Factors influencing the practice of community health nursing.

philosophy, similar to the dialects of any language, depending on factors such as local traditions of work, organizational differences, and so on. None of these variations could be dismissed as not the 'real' philosophy because that would assume an ideal against which any instance of practice could be measured. It is sometimes assumed that the public statements of professional theorists constitute just such a description of the ideal philosophy. However, these public statements are themselves merely selections and variations produced in the pursuit of particular goals. Neither is it true to say that any practice will directly correspond to the occupational philosophy. Any particular instance of practice will be a negotiation between occupational knowledge, the idiosyncratic personal knowledge and style of the practitioner and the client's expectations, values and beliefs (Fig. 1.1).

In order to illustrate this it will be useful to contrast three different types of account – official accounts, practitioners' accounts and teachers' accounts. To explore the construction of knowledge further it will be helpful to use Sharp and Green's (1975) description of the elements of an ideology which relates to the teaching profession. Thus ideology may be described as:

'A connected set of systematically related beliefs and ideas about what are felt to be the essential features of teaching. A teaching ideology involves both cognitive and evaluative aspects, it will include general ideas and assumptions about the nature of knowledge and of human nature – the latter entailing beliefs about motivation, learning and educability. It will include some characterisation of society and the role and functions of education in the wider social context. There will also be assumptions about the nature of the tasks teachers have to perform, the specific skills and techniques required together with ideas about how these might be acquired and developed. Finally the ideology will include criteria to assess adequate performance, both of the material on whom the teachers 'work', i.e., pupils, and for self-evaluation or the evaluation of others involved in educating. In short, a teaching ideology involves a broad definition of the task and a set of prescriptions for performing it, all held at a relatively high level of abstraction.' (Sharpe & Green, 1975 p. 68).

The four principles specified in 'An Investigation into the Principles of Health Visiting' (CETHV 1977) are:

(1)   search for health needs

(2) stimulation of the awareness of health needs
(3) influence on policies affecting health
(4) facilitation of health-enhancing activities

While these are expressed as 'principles' they clearly belong to Sharp and Green's category of a characterization of the role and functions of the occupation in the wider social context. These principles are related in the document to an underlying or more fundamental principle, namely that health is a valuable attribute, which is clearly a belief justifying the professional health visiting task. However, this belief is not presented in any context of other societal or personal goals. We are not told, for instance, if it is more valuable than education but less valuable than peace.

In accordance with Sharp and Green's definition, the health visiting principles are all expressed at a high level of abstraction. What is missing from the literature is a set of prescriptions for operationalizing these principles in terms of practical health visiting tasks, and the search for such prescriptions has been a matter for some reflection among health visitors. However, to an extent any abstract listing of prescribed tasks will be irrelevant to the complexities of practice.

We can contrast this official account with the practitioners' account as described in an ethnographic research study (Robinson, 1986). This research analysed audio-tape recordings of health visitors talking with clients during home visits to see how health visiting was constructed in practice. The study found that the home visits were highly organized encounters in which the practitioners took the leading role through, for example, deciding how long the visit would last, what sort of topics should be talked about, and who should talk about them.

An additional dimension can be added by Dingwall's study of health visitor training (Dingwall, 1977) in which he describes the sort of accounts or definitions of health visiting which health visitor tutors and fieldwork teachers passed on. For example, they emphasized the autonomy of each practitioner, and that the qualities of each practitioner are more important than skills. The importance of teachers' accounts will be explored in more detail in the next section.

It is important not to try to choose between such accounts or definitions, each of them is valid in a different way. The question 'what do community health nurses do?' may be answered by 'they think and act as community health nurses'. Any activity undertaken within a health visiting perspective could be a legitimate health visiting activity provided both the group and society legitimized it. Of central importance to a professional group is the need to control the members' perspectives, so that despite relative freedom from overt control, all members of the group only perform in ways that are likely to be seen as legitimate.

The segmentation of occupational knowledge

The discussion so far may have implied that occupational groups such as barristers, doctors and teachers, each embrace only one philosophy, albeit with dialects, to which all practitioners must subscribe. This is not necessarily the case. Any occupation may contain within it a number of subgroups, each of which will adhere to a different philosophy. Bucher and Strauss (1961) have called such subgroups 'segments' and they suggest that 'Different definitions may be found between segments of the profession concerning what kinds of work the profession should be doing, how work should be organized, and which tasks should have precedence. . .'. They illustrate their descriptions of occupational segments with reference to psychiatry, suggesting that: 'In psychiatry the conflict over the biological versus the psychological basis of mental illness continues to produce men who speak almost totally different languages. In recent years, the situation has been further complicated by the rise of social science's perspectives on mental illness.'

This reference to conflict in psychiatry in relation to three different scientific explanations of ill-health is interesting because it has been suggested that a similar conflict is being pursued in health visiting. According to the work of J. Robinson (1982) 'An Evaluation of Health Visiting' offers a wide vision of two major philosophies practiced by field level health visitors: the 'problem-oriented approach' and the 'relationship-centred approach'. In her view these two modes of practice are related to two distinct priorities for health visiting, each of which relies on a different theoretical structure. The problem-oriented approach is related to the screening techniques which are generated by the medical model of health. The relationship-centred approach is related to psychotherapeutic intervention techniques, which are derived ultimately from psychological notions of normal human growth and development. Robinson does not suggest that each philosophy (note that she calls them perspectives) is held to the exclusion of the other, but rather that in any situation they will come into play to differing degrees. In particular situations, she gives the example of the disposal of abnormal cases found by paediatric screening; health visitors may experience conflict as each philosophy emphasizes a different ideal course of action. Robinson's study is particularly concerned with the implications of these philosophies for the evaluation of health visiting (see Chapter 5). However, it is worth noting that the existence of these perspectives as practical occupational philosophies is as yet unexplored by empirical work. Their current status is that of hypothetical constructs 'based on the intuitive observation of health visitors at work, when relating to them in a managerial capacity' (Robinson, 1982 p. 29). In any case, such segmentation may have been altered by more recent emphasis on working with communities rather than individuals. Segments will prosper or decline in response to external as well as internal pressures.

THE ROLE OF TRAINING

Each segment of an occupation attempts to maximize its influence in the control of scarce resources. Influence over new entrants to the profession is particularly important because they constitute the 'new generation' of practitioners. This involves controlling the training, especially the syllabus, and the methods and practice of assessing the students. The segment which controls the passage into the profession may be able to promote its own definitions and prescriptions as the only acceptable ones, that is, the segment can ensure that its own version of the professional ideology predominates. Increasingly, control over research activity may also be valuable as this may focus attention on one aspect of work rather than another.

Dingwall (1977) provides us with a specific account of the presentation of occupational knowledge to students, and of their subsequent selection and organization of it, in his study of health visitor training courses. This account is central to any analysis of health visiting knowledge for reasons specified by Dingwall (1976). If, as he asserts, 'one of the key purposes of any training school is to transmit the knowledge which has to be drawn on by competent members of the occupation then one would expect to find the students being presented with a particularly explicit and formalized version of the occupational knowledge base. He suggests that this is especially likely in the case of health visiting because the private nature of much of health visiting work necessitates a more detailed and explicit socialization process if occupational conformity is to be ensured.

Dingwall found that the course concentrated on presenting the students with various theories of society. He says that the students' courses are intended to tell students explicitly or implicitly what their society is like (sociology, social policy and public health) and what individuals are like (psychology, child development, medical practice). He identified a number of different theorists encountered by the students; namely, the doctors, professional social theorists and official health visiting theorists, including both tutors and field staff.

The doctors' model, i.e. the medical model, is a predominant one in the National Health Service and therefore should be familiar to every health visitor student from her nurse training. It is part of the occupational ideology of the medical profession. It asserts an essentially mechanistic understanding of human beings which defines illness as the breakdown of a mechanism of the body in response to external physical forces or simple 'wear and tear'. (Thus the two responses of doctors to illness can be characterized as: 'there's a lot of it about' and 'it's your age.') The medical model defines an appropriate role for the doctor as super-mechanic, repairing the faulty part, and for the nurse as mechanic's assistant, performing simple diagnostic tests, undertaking prescribed remedies and keeping the machine in good order. This model is so pervasive in the health service that it may be held by health care workers at a subconscious level and not be seen as a model of health and illness but as 'the way things really are'. This is an example of a scientific theory which has diffused to the level of commonsense thinking as well as professional thinking.

The most influential of the professional social theorists propounded a version of social reality that Dingwall called the evangelical model. This social science model, which related both to psychology and sociology, presents to the students an 'expert' definition of how the social world functions and impinges on the individual; a model which is unavailable to the general public. It presents both an 'ideal' of personal and social functioning, which generates concepts of maladjustment related to current levels of sickness and health, and a selection of appropriate remedies to correct such maladjustment.

Dingwall also documents another contrasting professional social theory presented to the students, the latitudinarian model, which as the name suggests was not an expert version of reality but an analysis of other scientific and lay theories. Of the first two theories which offered 'expert' perspectives, Dingwall found that neither of them appeared particularly pertinent to the students, although Robinson's (1982) work suggests strongly that these theories may be found in practice. Dingwall (1977) suggests that the students did not adopt either model to the exclusion of the other. On the contrary, they were:

'... quite happy to invoke whatever theory seemed to be relevant in a given situation without regard to its consistency with any other theory that might be invoked on any other occasion.' (p. 84).

This leaves us with a major question. How is it that the student defines relevance *before* invoking the theory which will itself provide a definition of relevance? Dingwall implies two criteria for choice, based on the two characteristics of a social theory – its ability to formulate a version of society and to provide for the relevance of the theorist.

In order to see how students choose an appropriate model of society we must remember they bring with them to the course a whole range of practical commonsense theories about life. The presence of pre-existing models of life is irrelevant to many academic studies; biochemistry students, for instance, will have few theories on the structure and relationship of cells because that is not a field in which commonsense knowledge has very much to say. Community health nurses are, however, receiving tuition in the area in which commonsense lay knowledge is itself predominant, that is, social life and social relationships. Those subjects in which they receive tuition, such as family life, child care, normal development and the problems of ageing, are all areas in which they not only have some general knowledge but also some personal experience. The personal and commonsense knowledge of the student, therefore, will be focused on the same area as the new set of theories being presented to them. They do not therefore need to choose between the new theories according to scientific criteria; indeed as they are not scientists it is difficult to see how they could do so. Instead they use their existing commonsense theories to accept, reject or modify the new knowledge. Of course, their criteria will not necessarily be concerned with the impact of the theories in 'real life' but rather with the impact of the theories on the students' present concern, that is, getting through the course.

If we return to the second criterion for adopting or utilizing a theory, that it will provide a rationale for certain sorts of action, we can readily see that the evangelical model provides an understandable and sympathetic role for the health visitor. The evangelical model has precise definitions of what constitutes desirable social change and these usually involve practical social and personal changes. It is true that health visiting in practice concentrates on personal rather than social change but this may be as much a question of the structure of health visiting practice as philosophical choice. The medical model in contrast can only accommodate health visitors as subordinate personnel whose function is screening, surveillance, and the simple training of patients in routine procedures, all performed under the guidance or direction of the doctors. As a justification for practice, therefore, one would expect to find the evangelical model of a predictable social world, accessible only to expert understanding and amenable only to expert manipulation, to be successful as a part of health visiting philosophy regardless of its scientific merits as a system of explaining the social world.

Despite the direct presentation of different scientific versions of the world to his students by 'professional theorists', Dingwall observed that the accounts of life which the students found most relevant came from the 'official health visiting theorists', the tutors and field level staff. What were these accounts? The tutors' accounts (note that these are 'typical' constructs and do not specifically relate to any one tutor) were essentially psychologistic, that is, they utilized psychological explanations for social phenomena, although also combining elements of medical and sociological theories. Human nature was seen to be determined by the particular experience of the individual, especially childhood experiences. There were assumed to be 'normal' patterns of life related to one's age, class and gender, and maladjustment was construed as deviation from these norms. Dingwall notes that this view necessitated an individualistic approach to care, unlike the collectivist approach which was current at that time in hospital nursing practice which strove to achieve equality of care by treating patients equally rather than unequally. The accounts of the field level workers differed from those of the tutors by being less scientifically oriented and more moralistic. The central moral category was 'normal family life', a concept which was related to the circumstances of the family and in particular their social class categorization and social environment.

We conclude that the health visiting knowledge presented to the students did not consist of a series of 'facts' unrelated to anything the students might have had previous knowledge about. Instead it presented a range of material on subjects already familiar to the student. The implication is that the students' knowledge, being lay knowledge, is erroneous or at the least grossly parochial, and requires, in Dingwall's terms, 'new additions and revelations about social life'. This implication is already conveyed by placing the course in an institution of higher education rather than relying on the apprenticeship methods of nurse training.

Despite this overt orientation to scientific models, Dingwall suggests that the students were more impressed by the models presented by the field-work teachers. They used scientific models not as sufficient and independent explanations but as justifications reinforcing the validity of their existing moralistic models of society and of the value of health visiting intervention.

This dichotomy between the nature of professional knowledge and the means of its transmission is apparently not unique. Freidson (1977) has noted in relation to medical training that the formal educational structure related to an occupation may not correlate with the knowledge required for efficient productivity but exists as a means of classifying the status rather than the nature of the job. Similarly, a scientific method of transmitting knowledge may be required in preparation for an occupational role even though the knowledge being transmitted may not itself be scientific.

Knowledge in practice

So far we have presented a picture of occupational knowledge as the integral framework for guiding practitioners' actions. For example, the health visitor plans her routine visiting around particular age groups because her perspective on health incorporates age as a prime factor; she plans extra visits to single-parent families because of a perspective that establishes two parents as the norm and single parents as deviant. Her occupational knowledge is not a simple database but the organizing framework of all her health visiting actions and judgments: planning visits, writing records, talking to clients, talking to colleagues.

The community health nurse is not acting in a social vacuum but in a world busy with clients and colleagues, all of whom have their own perspectives, lay or professional. An occupational perspective has therefore to include strategies for negotiating and compromising with other perspectives in a situation of potential conflict, and especially notions of an integral core of knowledge which is the essential property of that particular occupation and is not open to negotiation.

The inevitability of conflict and the necessity of negotiation has not been adequately addressed in the nursing literature. Nurses are in general aware of the differences between lay and professional perspectives but these differences have not been explored in depth because they have been conceptualized, following the precedent of other health care settings, as problems of communication. Differences in perception which have been expressed in language or by client 'non-compliance' have been classified as simple problems of language use and interpretation which can be simply remedied by, for example, changing language styles.

However, it is more useful to see the meeting of different perspectives in practice as an arena of potential conflict and negotiation where each perspective is presented as the only 'real' view. We can then look at the sort of claims each negotiator uses to enhance their position and how unequal the participants may be in their willingness and ability to negotiate. In particular, the claim to professional status is intrinsically a claim for the superiority of the professional perspective which has implications for relationships with clients and colleagues. The discussions which follow will look in more detail firstly at the influence of a professional ideology in defining client problems and, secondly, suggest that inter-professional disputes may be the inevitable result of philosophical differences between colleagues.

Defining the client's problems

A most interesting example of the impact of professional definitions on the life of the client can be found in MacIntyre's (1976, 1977) work on the outcomes of pregnancy. Her study is based on observation of and interviews with a number of women throughout their pregnancy. MacIntyre found that there were essentially two models of appropriate action by which the women were being assessed by health workers, both models stemming from one professional theory on 'appropriate' child-bearing. The first model asserted that pregnancy and childbearing are normal and desirable and that to assume that they are problematic is wrong: that children should remain with their natural parents and the loss of a fetus or baby causes instinctive grief. The second presents a mirror image of the first. The desire for pregnancy and childbearing is abnormal and the state of pregnancy is problematic and requires special remedies; whereas a state of infertility does not; any child should be given up and the loss of a fetus or a child should not cause distress.

These two models are used contemporaneously because they are applied to different groups of women; the determining factor being whether the woman is married. MacIntyre found that the doctors based their judgment of the problems of the women largely on the single criterion of their actual or projected marital status. However, her account of the women's views of their own situation shows that their assessment of the desirable outcome of the pregnancy was not directly related to their marital status and they saw the two activities of marriage and childbearing not as necessary partners but as separate issues about which separate choices could and should be made.

MacIntyre herself raises the question of the position of the nurses:

'The majority of the nurses were female. However, partly because of its sex composition as well as its occupational tradition of service to 'the doctor', the nursing profession may give more credence to the theories of doctors than to those of women patients, and it may enhance its professional standing by allying itself to the medical profession and its body of knowledge. Nurses' theories about motherhood may, therefore, be informed more by those of clinicians than by their own experience or that of their female patients.' (MacIntyre, 1976; p. 156).

MacIntyre found, in addition, that in antenatal clinics the nurses were using the doctors' 'problem' categories by, for example, marking the notes of single women for special attention.

MacIntyre's work illustrates two further important issues. First, people can incorporate many theories into their lives and that some of these theories can be logically contradictory. MacIntyre tells us of a staff nurse who both castigates a single woman who is distressed at the loss of the fetus by spontaneous abortion as being immature and not fit to be a mother, and yet remarks later to the researcher that no woman is able to tolerate the loss of a fetus with equanimity. The nurse's remarks also serve to illustrate the second point.

Second, theories in application generate their own reinforcement. We can see how the 'immature' reaction of the unwed woman is 'evidence' that her pregnancy is not appropriate and of course the theory that it is not appropriate generates the label of immaturity in response to the distress. Similarly, MacIntyre illustrates that the special attention paid to the problems of unwed women generates increased data on their problems – thus 'proving' that they have more problems – whereas the problems of the married women were trivialized because it is 'known' that married women desire and enjoy pregnancy.

We are not concerned here with whether or not the professional theories described by MacIntyre are 'right' or whether they are in current use. The important issue here is the use of professional theory as a source of power over the client. All nurses will be familiar with conflict between professional and lay expectations in hospital where, for example, nurses attempt to mobilize patients as a matter of some urgency despite lay beliefs that sick people should stay in bed. In hospital it is relatively easy to control the patients' behaviour and to an extent patients expect their previous knowledge to be devalued – they are, after all, in a different 'world'. At home, however, people expect well understood, tried and tested knowledge to prevail as it is through this knowledge that their world is made understandable and amenable to their control. The professional attempt to replace this lay knowledge has serious consequences.

First, it may destroy confidence in lay knowledge and thereby create a vacuum. Second, the professional knowledge may impose oppressive definitions on the client. Third, to the extent that professional knowledge represents the needs of the state and acts as an agent of social control it may act in favour of particular dominant interests or classes to the detriment of others.

All three of these factors are exacerbated in the case of community health nursing knowledge because the majority of clients are women. The health of the family and care in time of sickness has traditionally been a forum of women's knowledge and the devaluation of such knowledge and its replacement by scientific knowledge must undermine the position of women and their confidence in their own private sphere of influence. The traditional routes for the transmission of such knowledge through the community and through the generations helped to forge links which were important to women, especially in times of trouble and during the difficult years of childbearing and childrearing. Practitioners discuss the decline of family ties but they themselves may be adding to the process by their denigration, implicit or explicit, of 'old wives' tales'.

Perhaps most of the criticism of the intrusion of professional knowledge into women's lives has come from the feminist movement which has drawn attention to the sexist nature of scientific definitions of human nature and in particular scientific definitions of health and illness (Brighton Women and Science Group, 1980). Because these definitions are based on science they are projected as women's biological destiny rather than social oppression, whereas they may simply be the expression of masculine definitions of women couched in scientific terms. Where these definitions are utilized by health care practitioners they can have a profound impact on women's lives, e.g. regulating their fertility, defining their dissatisfaction as 'mental illness', and judging their fitness to be mothers. This issue and its possible causes are addressed in an essay 'Feminism and Health Visiting' (Orr, 1982). Orr asserts that: 'Health Visitors as part of the wider society may enforce the values of a male dominated society, and their profession may reinforce these values because nursing (and health visiting) has a subservient relationship to the medical profession.'

There are many occasions when scientific knowledge is preferable to traditional remedies. An example is the treatment of children with a high temperature. Traditionally such children are kept warm but this may exacerbate their condition and cause febrile convulsions. It is therefore safer to lower the temperature of the child by tepid sponging, and practitioners are justified in promoting such remedies as superior to tradition. However, community health nursing is concerned with more than the advertisement of such simple remedies; it is concerned with making assessments about child care, normal child development, normal family life and the ageing process. Such assessments cannot be based on 'neutral' standards, however apparently scientific, because any such judgment must be intricately bound up with the social expectations of normality unique to British society in the latter half of the twentieth century. Orr cites the work of Comer (1974) to support this point when she argues that even assessments of normal child development are not merely biological but reflect the particular pattern of upbringing experienced by most British children; i.e. is a pattern of isolation for mothers and small children in the home which encourages certain sorts of behaviour and not others. Similarly, we have particular expectations of 'normal' behaviour in elderly people.

Defining relationships with colleagues

If we recall the two important consequences of adopting a professional philosophy; first that it will postulate the sort of society we live in and second, it will provide a particular 'role' for the professional worker, we can then see that conflict may arise when two different professional ideologies are brought to bear on any particular problem area. The workers may not agree on the dimensions of the problem, on whether it is a problem, on the appropriate action to take and who should take it. Take the example of child abuse: in any particular instance the workers involved may not agree whether it is abuse of a child or merely normal parental treatment. That is to say, although they may agree on what happened, i.e. that the child was hit, they may disagree about whether or not this was abnormal behaviour depending on their professional perceptions of family life and normal parental behaviour.

In the case of Lester Chapman, for example, there was no dispute that he was injured: the Report of the Inquiry (Reading, 1979) shows that the doctor observed 'about eight weals on the right buttock and three on the left, with the skin broken within some of the lesions'. The Inquiry was of the opinion that Lester should have been removed to a place of safety. However, most of the professionals who saw him had not taken that view. The detective sergeant is quoted as saying that if the same injuries had been inflicted upon a boy of thirteen by caning at school this would have been regarded as within the bounds of reasonable punishment. In this case, therefore, as in all others, the professional task was not to 'find' the truth, but to construct a reasonable account of the circumstances which involved judgments of what constitutes 'reasonable' punishment for a child at a particular age and inflicted by a particular adult.

Even if they agree that the child was abused they may have further difficulties over the cause. Is it, for example, individual 'wickedness' or the pressures of the environment, and should the perpetrator be punished or helped? If they are to be helped then they may not agree on the methods, e.g. using drugs or psychotherapy? Such conflicts can be both intra-professional and inter-professional, they can occur both between occupational segments and between occupations. In a study of the way in which health visitors and social workers identify and deal with child abuse (Dingwall, Eekelar & Murray, 1983) such differences are linked in part to the common experience of each of the types of workers. Social workers commonly deal with families in distress and difficulty and therefore develop a wider definition of 'normal' families than do health visitors whose primary role is to deal with families which are manifestly coping without intervention.

In a study of the different occupational structures and cultures of general practitioners and social workers, Huntington (1981) describes a number of 'ideal-type' practitioners. She outlines six 'ideal-type' general practitioners as follows:

(1) 'real doctor'
(2) father figure
(3) internal physician
(4) family doctor
(5) psycho-physician
(6) psychotherapist

She further describes four 'ideal-type' social workers:

(1) the caseworker as paramedical
(2) the caseworker as psychotherapist
(3) the generic social worker acting as change-agent at the micro-level
(4) the socialist social worker acting as change-agent at the macro-level

Although we have little empirical evidence, it is likely that many community health nurses could identify with one of the social worker 'ideal-types' outlined above.

These 'ideal-typical' constructs represent the different identities available to workers in each occupation, and Huntington suggests that in any general practitioner/social worker collaboration the 'match' between the two occupational identities may be an important factor in determining the ease or difficulty of the relationship. For instance, a general practitioner as internal physician could collaborate happily with a social worker as psychotherapist because their definitions of their respective roles are complementary. However, a general practitioner as a psycho-therapist would see such a social worker as a competitor. The socialist social worker acting as a change-agent at the macro-level would define medicine as oppressive and might find any collaboration with a doctor difficult. Obviously, this is not the only important factor in interoccupational differences, and Huntington attributes much importance to structural differences such as the different age and sex distributions in the professions. These structural differences almost certainly are important factors in the relationship between general practitioners and health visitors but they are difficult to change in the short-term. The relevance of cultural identities within occupations to intra-occupational collaboration could, however, be taken into account in policy-making.

This points the way to the importance of community health nurses understanding both their own philosophy and also general practitioners' philosophies, but also to examining the philosophies of their fellow nurses to see how nursing is divided into segments and how these segments accord with particular nursing tasks and responsibilities.

A number of authors have developed the theme that nursing can broadly be divided into the three segments of the managers, the professionalizers and the workers (see, for example, Carpenter, 1977). Currently, the professionalizers are clearly in the ascendant and have persuaded the occupation to adopt a number of innovations, such as the nursing process and primary nursing. Indeed the introduction of the pre-registration Diploma in Nursing and the increasing number of nursing degrees is evidence of their success. Their rise has been helped by the restructuring within the NHS which removed a number of nursing management layers and increased the emphasis on general rather than occupational management.

THE POLITICS OF HEALTH VISITING KNOWLEDGE

The status of nursing knowledge is currently being examined and redefined (Robinson & Vaughan, 1992). This is a consequence of the perception by nurses that the status of their knowledge is a factor in the competition for the finite resources of society such as money, status, independence and power. Here we discuss some of the limitations and consequences of nursing claims about nursing knowledge.

The roots of concern with occupational knowledge lie in the relationship between exclusive knowledge and professional power. Hitherto, professions have had the exclusive knowledge in particular areas of life. This monopoly can be used to benefit the occupation in arguments about resource allocation and policy-making; to define and control the client; and to organize, control and extend the area of work (Wilding, 1982).

Although there are other factors underpinning professional power, the prevailing strategy for occupational advancement is through the claim that the occupational perspective is unique, valid, specialized and abstract, and requires a long period of specialized education to master it. In modern industrial society the most powerful means of enhancing the status of knowledge is to associate it with science.

Schroyer (1971) has documented the claims made by what he terms 'prescriptive scientism'. These claims include the assertion that knowledge is essentially neutral, that it can be produced only by the scientific method, and that this method's standard of certainty and exactness is the only valid model. Thus knowledge is 'conceived of as a neutral picturing of fact' (Schroyer, 1971) and the consequences of this are far-reaching. Clearly if there is only one path to the 'true' view of any phenomenon then any scientist attempting to take a different view using a different method is 'in error' or a heretic, and any commonsense view is non-scientific and therefore by definition wrong. The scientist has become the high priest of knowledge admitting others only into roles as worshippers or heretics. This generates an unhealthy exclusivity in any democratic society, but it is particularly dangerous when the 'object' of study is the social world and scientific prescription involves the manipulation of individual human beings. Such manipulation is implicit, for instance, in some social skills training programmes based on behavioural science.

This notion of science providing the only route to the truth is a very influential ideology in nursing. McFarlane (1977), for example, cites Murphy's (1971) definition of the current body of knowledge in nursing as superstition, speculation and unrationalized experience and contrasts this with the preferred goal of a rational and scientific approach to nursing. The implicit assumption seems to be that all non-scientific knowledge is irrational and invalid, but this is not the case. The major part of life is conducted in a rational and sensible way. Virtually all the knowledge we have of our environment, of the weather, of the seasons, of food, of childcare, and of sickness and of health is derived from community traditions of knowledge rather than science. By and large, such knowledge has allowed us to manage our affairs very satisfactorily. Where particular areas of life have required specialized skills then they have been organized into crafts or fields of technological competence with a tradition of specialized organization and apprenticeship training. We think it is most useful to view community health nursing as one of these areas of specialization, related to, but not subservient to, scientific knowledge.

Knowledge and power are so closely interlinked, that the call to make nursing more scientific is essentially a political demand and is open to political discussion and comment. However, because the political strategy chooses an epistemological argument, that is, it bases its case on a claim about the status of its knowledge, it must also be open to epistemological objections. We will look first at the potential of nursing knowledge in comparison with other scientific knowledge, returning to the political questions at the end of the chapter.

The logical status of nursing knowledge

Nursing theorists pursue the chimera of nursing science with such vigour partly because they equate theorizing and rationality with science. As the ability to theorize and to act rationally is a human rather than an exclusively scientific trait, nursing theories can be perfectly rational and sensible without being scientific. We would go further and say that nursing theory cannot be scientific, because nurses' standards of rationality and purpose must be dictated by and be a product of nursing goals.

A scientific theory is descriptive and explanatory. It is not prescriptive in the sense that it says you should do X; it only indicates that if you do X, Y will inevitably follow, given a detailed set of conditions. The practical decision about whether Y is a desirable end, or whether it is possible to do Y given that you also want to do Z, is based on the occupational theory which relies on moral and utilitarian but not scientific criteria to make its judgments. It will say, for instance, that if Y = patient recovery then this accords with our occupational goals and we will adopt it as part of practice as far as is possible in the fluctuating environment in which nurses work. This is not an inevitable decision; in other philosophies at other times patient recovery may well be an undesirable end, as indeed it may be claimed to be with certain classes of severely handicapped patients.

Nursing theory is thus an occupational theory, or set of theories, which nurses employ in order to decide what to do as nurses. They may be rational and coherent, although not necessarily so, and they may be held in a subconscious form or they may be explicitly expressed. They are, however, not scientific; they arise from the needs of practice and are pragmatically validated in practice. There are a number of theories, both scientific and lay, which may be incorporated into these nursing theories in some form, for example, lay theories about male and female roles; scientific theories about human development. In addition there are also scientific theories of nursing derived from sociology which seek to understand nursing as a particular expression of social organization. The explanations offered by such theories may be of value to nursing in so far as nurses are prepared to use them to question their own conceptions of occupational practice. Occupational theories are therefore specialized theories produced by practitioners to account for their work and their problems. They are the main organizing force of practice and the matrix through which both scientific and lay theories are filtered.

The political implications of changing nursing knowledge

We have described how the nursing claim to a scientific knowledge framework is invalid. However, a claim does not have to be valid to succeed. The claim of doctors to have a scientific knowledge base is a very powerful factor in reinforcing their status, despite evidence that medicine is not scientific in practice (Huntington, 1981). An obvious example of the absence of scientific rationality would be found in the numerous studies of the differential rates of particular types of surgery between different countries (there is a useful discussion in Open University 1985a Chapter 7, and 1985b, Chapter 3). Of course, the surgeons' decisions may be entirely rational in commonsense terms – the figures seem to be related in part to the financial reward systems operating in the various countries!

Unfortunately, those seeking to use medicine as a precedent have misunderstood the link between medical knowledge and medical power. The unique historical conditions which created the major monopolistic professions are unrepeatable. Aspiring professions are no longer attempting to 'expand into a fluid market situation but into areas of highly organized, legally protected and entrenched professional interests. Freidson (1975) argues that there is no room for further professionalization in the health services because of the pre-eminence of the medical profession. However, although re-organizing the occupational philosophy may not be a thoroughly successful strategy it may exacerbate the problems in the relationships with clients and colleagues discussed earlier. In particular it will reduce the power and control exercised by the client. As Freidson comments:

'Faith, which all men (*sic*) may possess, and politics, in which all citizens of a democratic country may participate, fade away before knowledge which only experts possess. Decisions requiring expertise are insulated from the public debate, negotiation and compromise that is politics; faith in revealed dogma or in a given set of morals is declared out of order. Laymen are excluded from participating in decisions thought to require special expertise, even when those decisions are intended to improve their own well-being' (Freidson, 1975 p. 335).

In so far as any occupational group claims to have special knowledge, unavailable to any other worker or to the client, and amenable only to evaluation by that group, it is excluding all others from the power to describe, define and control an area of life. An example of such an exclusion, backed by law, is the case of legal judgment against any lay organization of childbirth without medical assistance. Imagine the same principles in action in community health nursing practice: weaning your child before the age of four months is illegal; failure to attend the clinic regularly incurs heavy fines; the practitioner has the right to enter any home. Such powers might seem absurd, and few would seek them, yet that is what the possession of an exclusive body of knowledge implies – the expert is right and the client is wrong. We already structure nursing language in this fashion, talking of the non-compliant client and the non-attender at clinic. It may be that the influence of the nurse is always a force for good, although we doubt it, and that the power of the state expressed through the actions of the nurse is essentially benevolent. There are some obvious areas where this is usually the case, such as the protection of the rights of a child against a neglectful or abusing parent. The important concern here, however, is that by expressing and justifying such power in scientific rather than moral terms, the professional activities are protected from political debate and non-professional examination. 'Life' issues, such as how to bring up your children and what to eat, are transformed into technical questions susceptible only to technical expertise. Zola (1972) offers the debate over fluoridation as an example of a political question being turned into a scientific question. He says the argument is easier to win when it is removed from the democratic to the public health arena; from the arena of opinion and choice to that of scientific 'fact'.

However, before leaving this chapter it might be helpful to reiterate the important themes and then to emphasize the limitations of the discussion. Themes which we hope you will be able to utilize in your future reading are, first, that knowledge is a dynamic process which is continuously produced, applied and tested through use. Second, that knowledge is a resource which is differentially distributed in society and which has a relationship with social power, influence and control.

The final caveat with which we will end is that we currently have insufficient knowledge of community health nursing practice and the perspectives which are in everyday use. Although we consider that examples of research into the perspectives of other health workers and occupations are interesting and often illuminating for nursing, it would be helpful to have a store of evidence about health practice in all its variations from which to draw examples and illustrate arguments. The major route to have such information is an increase in research activity.

2   The Community Dimension

Jean Orr

HEALTH AND COMMUNITY

As we approach the year 2000 there is an increasing emphasis on the relationship between health and community. Within the context of health care, the understanding of the concept of community is central to the delivery and focus of health care for all health care professionals and community nurses in particular. In many ways, health visitors have led the field in the importance and emphasis which was put on the idea of community. In 1977, for example, the Council for the Education and Training of Health Visitors' Principles Document (CETHV, 1977) defines health visiting in terms of assessing and meeting the health needs of the individual, the family and the community. Within the past decade the focus of education for community nurses has stressed the importance of working at a community level.

Within the National Health Service and Community Care Act 1990 the District Health Authorities are expected to assess the health needs of the resident population and purchase services to meet the needs from the providers of service. For the first time, the health needs of the population should in theory be the rationale for the care provided. In this scenario community nurses will be in a prime position to assist in the compilation of data for districts, providing not only a range of quantitative data but also a wealth of qualitative data on the communities and populations they serve. The difficulty will be in health visitors having access to the planning mechanism at district level in order to feed in the data.

A definition of health

Health is described in the preamble of the Constitution of the WHO (1946) as 'a state of complete physical, mental and social well being, not merely the absence of disease or infirmity'. This definition is now being criticized because it describes an ideal state rarely attained in the real world. A more useful definition is that of the Ottawa Charter for Health Promotion:

'Health is created and lived by people within the settings of their everyday life; where they learn, work, play and love. Health is created by caring for oneself and others, by being able to take decisions and have control over one's life circumstances, and by ensuring that the society one lives in creates conditions that allow the attainment of health by all its members'. (WHO, CPHA 1986)

This definition places health firmly in the context of community. The context of prevention can have a negative image, and often embodies the notion of discouraging persons from doing things that will harm them. Now the thrust in many countries is towards the positive concept of health maintenance and promotion; not merely prevention. This concept aims to encourage all inhabitants to lead healthful lives and includes eating healthful diets, exercising regularly and maintaining a positive outlook on life with due regard for regular periods of rest and relaxation. Health promotion is viewed as a process of enabling people to increase control over and to improve their health. It represents an attempt to move from planning medical care services to planning for healthy people and healthy environments, and nurses involved in any health care have a vital role to play in prevention and health promotion, as do a wide range of others such as town planners, environmental health officers, etc.

The subject of prevention should be viewed in the global context embodied in the goal of the World Health Organisation (WHO, 1981) 'Health for All by the Year 2000'. All member states of WHO attending the world health assembly agreed that the main social target of governments and of WHO should be the provision of some form of health care that would be accessible to all citizens regardless of where they lived: in remote villages; in rotting urban cores, etc. Although one might concur that the idea of 'Health for All by the Year 2000' is not a realizable goal in many of the developing and some of the developed countries of the world, this target – often referred to as the WHO slogan – has provided incentives for national and international health planners and policy makers. WHO reports that progress is being made towards improved health that would not have otherwise taken place had this target not been enunciated and accepted as a goal by all governments of the world.

Recent trends in primary health care

The trend in primary health care has been to involve the community in the planning and delivery of health care. This makes explicit a shift in the relationship between the professional health workers and the community. It is envisaged that local people will be encouraged by the professionals to take a more active role in health care issues. For example, in 1974, the World Health Organisation (WHO, 1974) defined community nursing not only as including family health nursing but as also being concerned with identifying the community's broad health needs and involving the community in development projects related to health and welfare. Community nursing is said to be involved in helping communities to identify their own problems, to find solutions, and to take such actions as they can before calling on outside assistance. This would be in keeping with the views expressed in the Principles Document (CETHV, 1977).

Within the World Health Organisation there has been a gradual shift of emphasis in primary health care to include the recipients of care in planning. The changes in public and professional opinion were set forth in the Declaration of Alma Ata (WHO, 1978). They can be summarized under four headings:

(1)   Health care should be related to the needs of the population.
(2)   Consumers should participate, both individually and collectively, in the planning and implementation of health care.
(3)   The fullest use must be made of available resources.
(4)   Primary health care is not an isolated approach but the most local part of a comprehensive health system.

In 1981 when the World Health Organisation adopted 'Health for All by the Year 2000' as a global strategy, the aim was that by 2000 all peoples in all countries should have at least such a level of health that they are capable of working productively and of participating actively in the social life of the community in which they live. The three main objectives of the strategy are as follows:

(1)   Promote healthy lifestyles.
(2)   Prevent preventable conditions.
(3)   Enable the rehabilitation of those whose health has been damaged.

Within Europe this strategy has led to the 33 member countries agreeing to a set of 38 targets as steps on the path to 'Health for All by the Year 2000'. It is important to emphasize that the countries involved agreed to take forward these aims. We should also note that these objectives are the aims of health visiting and community nursing.

The more recent nursing discussion paper on 'Targets for Health for All' (WHO, 1986) develops the theme further and states that:

(1)   Health for all implied equity - that is that everyone should have access to health and health services.

(2)   The aim is to help people build and maintain health and therefore the emphasis is on prevention of disease and the promotion of health.
(3)   The people will achieve health for all and need to be well informed, well motivated and given the chance to actively participate in the process.
(4)   Co-operation is necessary with other sectors of Government as health is influenced by social and economic factors.
(5)   Lastly, the centre of the Health Care System should be primary health care.

The WHO discussion paper says that as advocates for the community, nurses will help in the essential task of involving the people in making decisions about health care and speak for the people's interest in the health care system and in political, economic and social decision making. Despite the many statements about health and health promotion it is still the case that most monies and personnel go to the acute sector and most decisions about the deployment of nursing resources are made at the centre. Job descriptions for health visitors, for example, do not normally vary according to the characteristics and circumstances of local populations.

It is to be hoped that changes in nursing education, namely through Project 2000, will give a new health focus to nurses; at present, however, nurses, doctors and other health personnel are educated to care for the sick and the larger majority of highly skilled personnel remain in sickness-orientated institutions. In many countries, the vast majority of all 'health workers' are devoting all their time to less than 5% of the population who are in hospitals on any given day. This militates against the achievement of the 'Health for All' goal; it must be pursued by governments who allocate the 'health' money, by educators who prepare the practitioners for the 'health' services, and by citizens who press for health programmes that are accessible. In addition, nurses, because of their sheer numbers, can press for changes in the 'sickness' system where the doctor is the gatekeeper. In most countries, only 5%-15% of nurses work in the community setting (Mussallum, 1988).

In a recently published document, *Achieving Health for All: A Framework for Health Promotion* (Epp, 1986), it is proposed that achieving health for all entails three challenges, three health promotion mechanisms and three implementation strategies, as follows:

(1)   Health challenges: reducing inequities in the health of low versus

Table 2.1 Focus of 'Targets for Health for All' by the year 2000 in Europe (WHO, 1986)

Targets 1-12: Health for all

1 Equity in health
2 Adding years to life
3 Better opportunities for the disabled
4 Reducing disease and disability
5 Eliminating measles, polio, neonatal tetanus, congenital rubella, diphtheria, congenital syphilis and indigenous malaria.
6 Increased life expectation at birth
7 Reduced infant mortality
8 Reduced maternal mortality
9 Combatting disease of the circulation
10 Combatting cancer
11 Reducing accidents
12 Stopping the increase in suicide

Targets 13-17: Lifestyles conducive to health for all

13 Developing healthy public policies
14 Developing social support systems
15 Improving knowledge and motivation for healthy behaviour
16 Promoting positive health behaviour
17 Decreasing health-damaging behaviour

Targets 18-25: Producing healthy environments

18 Policies for healthy environments
19 Monitoring, assessment and control of environmental risks
20 Controlling water pollution
21 Protecting against air pollution
22 Improving food safety
23 Protecting against hazardous wastes
24 Improving housing conditions
25 Protecting against work-related health risks

Targets 26-31: Providing appropriate care

26 A health care system based on primary health care
27 Distribution of resources according to need
28 Re-orientating primary medical care
29 Developing teamwork
30 Co-ordinating services
31 Ensuring quality of services

Targets 32-38: Support for health development

32 Developing a research base for health for all
33 Implementing policies for health for all
34 Management and delivery of resources
35 Health information systems
36 Training and deployment of staff
37 Education of people in non-health sectors
38 Assessment of health technologies

high income groups, increasing the prevention effort, enhancing people's capacity to cope.

(2) Mechanisms intrinsic to health promotion: encouraging self care to inspire healthy choices, mutual aid, creation of healthy environments.

(3) Strategies: fostering public participation, strengthening community services, co-ordinating public policy.

It is important to look at some of the reasons why preventive health services are difficult to get on the national agenda. First, it seems that the more privatized the health care system the less emphasis is put on prevention. Second, the medical dominance of health care systems means that prevention gets a low priority, especially if it is carried out by nurses. Third, health visiting is a service largely for women by women and as such may not be seen as important by the policy makers. In a report, *Women, Health and Development* (WHO, 1985) the authors outline the major problems facing women and stated that women carry extra responsibilities for health through their contribution to the health of their families and communities, both formally and informally.

This preponderance of women in health care activities is true for most countries, developing and developed, and is a phenomenon which predates the emergence of modern health care systems. It is the women who are expected to be health educators; to teach sound health practices to future generations; to create a home environment that is conducive to health (from the provision of clean water to nutritious food); to limit family size; to ensure that children are immunized and cared for during crucial years and to take them to the formal health care services when necessary; and to care for the elderly. They constitute the majority of volunteers in hospitals, self-help clinics, and other community organizations. They are, therefore, already providing a giant's share of primary health care and yet women are expected to fulfil these multiple roles while being the least educated and informed members of society, as outlined by the WHO report *Having a Baby in Europe* (WHO, 1984).

The community health nursing partnership

A framework for primary health care which challenges present practice has been devised by Bergman (1981). The community is described as the main resource and focus of practice, and is to be in continuous interaction and communication with the primary health care worker, i.e. the nurse. The goal of community partnership is to help people reach, as far as possible, a state of self-reliance.

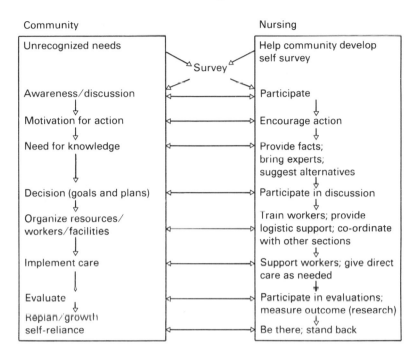

Fig. 2.1. Community nursing partnership in primary health care. From *Regional Workshop on Nursing and Midwifery Personnel in Primary Health Care*, Manila, 1979. Reprinted by permission of the World Health Organisation.

Colliere (1981) stressed the importance of fitting into the existing work situation rather than making the situation fit our preconceptions. Nurses should learn about the clients' ideas and use the clients' experience as the first source of knowledge. Primary health care relies on a new concept of health influenced by biological, cultural, social, economic and political factors. These factors are seen to be interrelated. Writing about the development of primary health care in an earlier paper, Colliere (1980) says that nurses should be prepared to work with the population and not for the population. This requires a change in the nurse/client relationship moving away from the provider/recipient model. While these ideas of partnership may be new to us they are equally new to the clients and the community. Little discussion takes place about how we can involve the community and how we can motivate people to join in the decision-making process. As a result, health visiting finds itself in a dilemma. On the one hand health visitors are being encouraged to develop a community dimension which has a participative aspect, and on the other hand they have little guidance as to what form this should take and the issues involved. One of the main questions remains, what do we mean by participation and the issues involved?

Citizen participation – what is it?

Citizen participation has been taken to signify the right of citizens to ensure adequate delivery of services and to have a say in deciding what these services should be. The Seebohm Committee (HMSO, 1968) saw participation in the social services as:

(1) A place where people are engaged in providing services or help.
(2) Contribution to the decision-making process.
(3) Participation in the form of pressure groups publicizing needs or shortcomings in provision.

Participation, in this example, is put forward in terms of assumed consensus of interest, consensus between decision-makers and the public, and throughout the public itself. A more realistic view of participation centring on the decision-making process is presented by Arnstein (1969). Here participation is seen as 'the redistribution of power that enables the "have not" citizens presently excluded from the political and economic processes to be deliberately included in the future'. Arnstein examines participation by representing levels of involvement on what she calls a ladder of participation. The bottom rungs of the ladder are 'manipulation' and 'therapy' which are used to describe levels of non-participation which have been sometimes used to substitute for genuine participation. Often these strategies are used to educate or cure the participants. The next rungs involved 'informing' and 'consulting' without necessarily heeding what is said.

The following level of participation allows participants the right to 'advise' although not to make decisions. These levels represent various degrees of tokenism, and the top three rungs of the ladder are seen as 'partnership', 'delegated power' and finally 'citizen control' and represent true participation. Gilbert (1972) suggests that there are three types of participation, namely:

(1) Pseudo participation, which makes no perceptible change.
(2) Tokenism, where there is client influence on decision-making but only to a degree that makes very little practical difference.
(3) Redistributive participation, where clients are able to exert influence on decision-making.

We can see similarities with Arnstein's analysis in that it is assumed that a system which has redistributive participation will be more responsive to client needs them a system where decision-making is reserved only for professionals. The criticism can be made that these writers assume a homogeneity which may not exist among the 'have nots'. Both writers, however, do place questions about the role and degree of participation in the context of political power. In terms of outcome, participation often delivers less than it promises for the following two reasons. The area of involvement may be limited to safe issues, reinforcing existing social and political attitudes and curtailing the field of discussion. Secondly, in order to get participation, groups may have to reduce their demands.

Groups may be forced to change the pattern of their activities in such a way that they cease to pose any substantial challenge. The alternative for the group may be to find itself ignored totally. In this way, non-established organizations sometimes lose if they participate and lose if they do not. Examples of this can be seen in many tenants' associations campaigns where groups settle for less than they really want in order to gain something. This is highlighted by Dearlove (1974) who argues that authorities are able to control and regulate groups and are keen for groups to assume roles that help authorities to provide services for which there is an established demand. Failing this, the authorities are happy if groups assume a self-help role so that they can provide services without public funds. Is this also true of the National Health Service? Numerous groups absorb the ethos of self-help or else are realistic enough to see the difficulty of moving Government and assume an undemanding role from the start, thus reducing or avoiding conflict.

Client involvement in the National Health Service

The extent of client participation in the National Health Service is minimal. The ethos of the service stems from the early public health movement which believed that community participation was necessary to help eradicate communicable disease but the participation could only be under the guidance of the health care professionals. At present, therefore, the medical/health professionals are dominant because it is believed that they have the capacity and technology to improve health. The curative aspects are emphasized at the expense of preventive health care and social or economic change.

Moran (1991) sets out some concerns about the outcomes of the NHS and Community Care Act (1990). These concerns reflect the inherent difficulties of reconciling public health approaches with a market-led health care system. Firstly, he sees the NHS hospital trusts as having little interest in public health since this would require both a cost in itself and, if successful, actually reduce patient admission and attendances and hence hospital income.

Secondly, as large areas of the health service are to become shrouded in 'commercial confidentiality', collaboration and public accountability will inevitably decrease. The new hospital trusts are required to meet in public only once a year to present their business plan. Thirdly, the reforms will make short-term goals and contracts paramount and may have little interest in the long-term ideas of participation. While the new system may offer welcome encouragement to the expansion of individual consultation through patient satisfaction surveys, participation at a strategic level will be a problem. Fragmentation, reduced formal represent-ation, greater secrecy, and confusion about the consultation proce-dures will present serious obstacles to voluntary and community groups with limited resources. Moran welcomes the restatement of the role of the community health councils as public representatives. He is con-cerned that they will have no new statutory powers or enhanced funding to enable them to respond to the more complex structures.

Finally, to stress public participation is seen as threatening in so far as it suggests that the goodwill of professionals or bureaucratic rationality are insufficiently reliable to secure responsiveness to client needs. It also recognizes that the client and the organization have multiple objectives, and that in each case their own survival is foremost.

Issues of participation

In the field of health care there are different views about how the public can participate. These differences focus on four major questions about public involvement, as follows:

(1)   Who speaks for the community?
(2)   What changes will occur in client/professional relationship?
(3)   What organizational developments are needed?
(4)   How can the client be encouraged to participate?

Who speaks for the community?

In practice, client participation requires the election of appointment of one or more representatives. Many people do not have the time or the interest to participate in the making of every decision that affects them. It is necessary to face the issues of which clients participate, on whose behalf they participate and how they are chosen?

Many attempts to select representatives lack any formal accountability mechanisms to ensure that the opinions and objectives of participants are valid expressions of the local community. This is a problem experienced also in obtaining representatives to trade unions and professional bodies. This could result in community control becoming control of the community by some elements to the exclusion of others (Kenner, 1986). There is a danger that an elite group of activists could monopolize the attempts to achieve participation; this was found by Butcher *et al.* (1980) who surveyed five groups set up under the Community Development Project. All five displayed varying degrees of elitism and this characteristic persisted over time. It would be unrealistic to assume that all groups within the community share the same values and beliefs and have the same needs. There may be a number of people within a community whose needs are not articulated or acknowledged. For example, it is possible that drug addicts or pregnant teenagers may not have their needs articulated by community representatives who do not wish to recognize their existence because of the stigma involved.

What changes will occur in client/professional relationship?

The shift in emphasis to client involvement forces us to question our beliefs about the extent to which lay people are capable of understanding and implementing activities which have traditionally been the domain of trained professionals. The professional domination in the field of health care results from the withholding of knowledge and limiting access to resources.

Information is power and from that stems income and status, with ensuing social, political and economic consequences. Freidson (1977) says that as a result of this a class of people with specialized training and standard certifications have been able to serve a growing and, in part, self-created demand for their skills. This means that these professionals monopolize major decisions about how wealth, resources and skills are used. It is therefore possible to see why resources are directed to prestige projects and withheld from 'unpopular' client groups such as the elderly and mentally handicapped.

Health care professionals often resent alternative strategies for delivering care and one example of this is the setting up of well women's clinics. In some instances the professionals exhibit hostility and question the existence of the need for such a service even when this need has been documented (Orr, 1987). Clients' needs are often determined by professional skills in that it tends to be institutional imperatives which determine the validity of clients' problems and which professional should deal with these.

What organizational developments are needed?

How can we create and maintain suitable organizations to support any level of participation? In what ways can the public become involved both on an individual and group basis to make a necessary contribution to health care? In this issue there is an inherent tension between the need to institutionalize activities in order to ensure stability and the necessity to maintain flexibility and be responsive to changing local needs.

How can the client be encouraged to participate?

We need to recognize that participation will have costs, both economic and social, and may initially be resisted. Do we understand what motivates individuals to participate and what factors will facilitate collective action by a community?

In a study of self-help initiatives in inner London boroughs, it was found that the poor did not organize themselves into groups spontaneously. The groups depended on the leadership of articulate and forceful individuals who on their own admission were 'middle class professionals with the confidence to air their opinions' (Knight & Hayes, 1981).

The poor do not organize themselves (Pahl, 1970) for three reasons. Firstly, community group activities have to compete with other aspects of the social, political and spiritual life of an individual. Secondly, adjustment to problems tends to be individualistic, especially in situations of high housing mobility or among newcomers to housing estates. There will be no desire for collective action unless there is a common objective. Thirdly, deprivation itself inhibits the social action of the deprived. It is also difficult to start new ventures when these are dependent on external funding. The need for audits, annual reports and written applications requires participants who are literate, numerate and politically sophisticated. The cost to an individual will be high in terms of time, energy and possibly money (Hirsch, 1977). Just as we may scapegoat a patient who does not attend for what we see as acceptable treatment we may blame people for not organizing when the costs of doing so are simply too great and the structure of the service makes participation difficult.

We can see that there are considerable problems in moving to a participative model and as yet we have barely begun to turn the rhetoric into reality. If we are to embrace community participation it is essential that we have an understanding of what is meant by the term community, and in the chapter that follows we examine possible models of participation.

A NEW DEFINITION OF COMMUNITY

Much confusion seems to surround the usage of the term community. This occurs despite the fact that the notion of a community is central to the provision of health care and to the description of social life in general. It can be agreed that of all the concepts in terms of which we characterize, organize and constitute our social and political experience that of community is the most neglected (Plant, 1978). The various meanings and confusion surrounding the concept community occurs because the word is used both in descriptive and evaluative terms. Just think of the many ways we use the word: we talk of community nursing, community spirit, community policing, the European Community, community education and so on. In addition, when the term community is used it often not only describes a range of features in social life but puts these features in a favourable perspective. It is suggested by Greer and Minar (1969) that community refers to a unit of society and to aspects of that society which we value. Unlike many other terms in relation to social organization, such as state or society, the term community is seldom used in an unfavourable context.

Benson (1976) reinforces this view when he says the word is often used in a strongly evaluative and emotive way. For example, when we talk of community spirit the implication is that this is somehow a 'good thing'. When we talk like this we are not referring to an objectively definable type of social structure, instead we are referring to a vaguely sensed and worthwhile quality of common life which is felt to be valued and is assumed to depend for its existence on a specific type of social structure, such as a small village.

Within the concept of community, however, there are negative connotations. By defining an 'in group' making up a community we are, by implication, identifying an 'out group' of those who do not belong. One has only to think of Ulster, Brixton or Toxteth where such a phenomenon exists. Furthermore, the existence of a community can result in the use of informal means of social control being exerted to maintain community norms and values.

Updating the meaning of 'community'

Many words have both evaluative and descriptive meaning. A word such as 'beautiful', for example, can be used in both ways. It is necessary therefore to be aware of the confusion which can arise with these two kinds of meanings. We must be clear about which descriptive features of a social group are relevant to the value judgments that are made of it.

Some words touch on so many diverse phenomena depending on the context in which they are used (Tucker, 1979). Community is such a word because it is prone to multiple connotations and therefore misunderstandings. The term is frequently used both verbally and in writing with the assumption that there is a shared sense of meaning: 'community care', for example, is talked and written about as if there was total agreement among professionals as to its meaning. Such assumptions lead to confusion and make it necesary to formulate a working definition of this term. In so doing it is essential to examine some of the issues involved. Such a definition will, and should, be open to debate within nursing. It may be useful therefore to begin by examining some of the attempts which have been made to define what is meant by community.

The word community has been in common usage since its Latin origin as *communitas*. There are no less than 100 definitions available for the *communis* from which this word was derived (Weaver, 1977). Hilary (1955) articulated the problems involved when attempting to define the word. One of the major difficulties is the enormous number of contexts and structures to which the term has been applied. It has been used to describe geographical areas and linked to similar concepts like locality and neighbourhood. It describes ethnic links, e.g. the Jewish community, and describes functional links, e.g. a community of Masons.

Hilary (1955) re-examined 94 definitions and found that the most significant areas of agreement among 20 of the definitions were about the 'possession of common ends, norms and means'. The idea of life in common appeared in nine of the definitions, self-sufficiency in eight and consciousness of some kind in seven.

In attempting to analyse the word community further, Tonnies (1887) contrasts the concepts of *Gemeinshaft* and *Gezellschaft*. *Gemeinshaft* is described as the most basic form of human grouping characterized by rich and satisfying relationships. *Gezellschaft* on the other hand describes those relationships which are essentially superficial and impersonal. When interpreting Tonnies' view in the light of 20th century values, McIver and Page (1961) describe community as an area of social living marked by some degree of social coherence. The bases of community therefore are locality and community sentiment. The Seebohm Committee (HMSO, 1968) stated that a community can be held to exist if members have relationships which are reciprocal and ensure mutual aid and if the members experience a sense of well-being.

Midwinter (1973), on the other hand, sees a community as being an abstract entity, yet one which most people see themselves as belonging to. Newby and Bell (1971) see definitions of community as implying the organization of people, goods, services and commitments in a specific area with a marked emphasis upon sharing both the common good and the locality. Konig (1968) reinforces this view in claiming that in a strictly sociological sense the phenomenon of spatial proximity of neighbourhood is inseparable from the idea of community. An example of this concept is seen in Weiner (1975) when he studied the fragmentation of a community in the Shankhill area of Belfast. He described the community as a hierarchical structure, beginning with the extended family, moving through street collectives to the whole entity which he described as the Shankhill community. His concern was with the sets of relationships which existed in the area and to which inhabitants attributed great value. This prescriptive use of the word community implies that certain sets of relationships are valued as worthwhile in that they constitute a community.

A useful re-examination of the concept of community analyses the literature under the following headings:

(1)   Community as locality
(2)   Community as social activity
(3)   Community as social structure
(4)   Community as sentiment

The essential elements are identifiable as being a sense of solidarity, a sense of significance and a sense of security (Clark, 1973). The sense of sentiment is similar to what McIver and Page (1961) call the 'we-feeling'. They define this as 'the feeling that leads men to identify themselves with others so that when they say "we" there is no thought of distinction and when they say "ours" there is no thought of division'. Clark says that solidarity is by far the most commonly accepted ingredient of community and it is this sentiment which writers have in mind when they refer to social unity, togetherness, social cohesion and a sense of belonging.

The sense of significance is similar to what McIver and Page term 'role-feeling'. They define this as 'a sense of place or station experienced by group members so that each person feels he has a role to play, his own function to fulfil in the reciprocal exchanges of the social scene'. The sense of security is what McIver and Page call 'dependency-feeling'. They see this as involving physical dependency and psychological dependency, but Clark (1973) maintains that this sense of security comes from a sense of solidarity. If it is accepted that a sense of solidarity and a sense of significance are the two essential indicators, then Clark proposes the following working definition. The strength of community within any given group is determined by the degree to which its members experience both a sense of solidarity and a sense of significance within it. Clark sees this meaning resulting in a major re-orientation of approach in that the emphasis must be on how the members of the group themselves feel. This is not to argue that other more general sociological indices are of no consequence. What is proposed is that any investigation of community must begin by finding out how people feel about the community and not rely on the patterns of social activity, norms, roles and status systems.

The Barclay Report (1982) on social work reflects this emphasis on being where the people are, and says that:

> 'Community is a word with many meanings. What we mean is best illustrated from the standpoint of an individual living in a particular locality. He is likely to share some things in common with, and to feel some loyalty towards a number of other people within a particular geographical area - his family, his immediate neighbours, relatives and friends. . . . More remote but important for his peace of mind are local representatives and officials who determine his rates, clear his rubbish'.

The report goes on to talk about the many networks of relationships which are important for people, particularly if they are in trouble and need information, practical help, understanding or friendliness. It is these local networks of informal and formal relationships, together with the capacity to mobilize individual and collective responses to adversity, that the report sees as being one of the ways in which the word community is used. By this is meant the range of relationships which an individual may have outside a geographical area. These relationships may revolve around work or leisure activities, friends who live far away or the existence of a mutual handicap or political activity; the allegiance to these networks outside the local area may be as important or more important emotionally than the networks based on spatial considerations alone.

Classifying communities: two approaches

Any attempt to classify communities invariably draws from two approaches. The first utilizes objective data to measure the nature of community and the conditions of life in it. Measures referred to as objective depend on events or objects that can be counted and require little personal evaluation from the reporting individual. The second utilizes subjective data which comes directly from the perceptions, evaluations and opinions of people concerning the condition of life in their communities. An example of an objective measure of safety might be the number of reported crimes in an area. A subjective approach to measuring safety might be to ask local people whether they feel safe going out. While this distinction is a useful and relevant one, the difference between objective and subjective data is not always clear. The crime figures, for example, will be a feature of what information is recorded and what crimes go unreported.

These two orientations are complementary rather than competing systems of description. Each may be relevant to differing kinds of behaviour and it is the interaction between these two which may help us to understand the community. Satisfaction with where we live is, after all, not just based on factors such as housing standards and educational facilities - important as these may be. We also possess feelings and sentiments about the area in which we live.

Subjective data

The subjective elements go to make up what has been called the social climate which affects the quality of life (Moos, 1976). Moos suggests that environments have unique personalities just as people do. Some are supportive, some competitive. This approach, using the environmental-social, rather than the environmental-physical, emphasizes impressionistic elements of description.

Historically, planners and policy makers have placed their reliance on objective measures of a community. They have measured such things as housing and unemployment because it is argued that such factors influence people's lives. These types of measures are useful because they enable comparisons to be made between areas and groups and can be a guide to changing socio-economic conditions. The question, however, remains as to the meaning of these statistics and their relationship to the subjective experience. We can, for example, measure the housing density but what does that tell us about the pleasures or problems of living in a particular estate? According to Campbell *et al.* (1976) the use of social indicators alone is not sufficient, and in order to know the quality of life experiences one must go directly to the individual for a description of what life is like. Krupat and Guild (1980) examined a number of factors which they suggest could be used to capture the social climate of a city or community. Six meaningful factors emerged by which social climate can be described. These are:

(1) *Warmth and closeness.*
This first and most important factor contains items reflecting general feelings of security and support which an environment may provide such as: relaxed atmosphere, sense of intimacy, a safe, healthy and peaceful place and friendly people.

(2) *Activity and entertainment.*
This contains items such as: activity, entertainment, diverse selection, dense population, and an atmosphere of culture. Density is seen as being related to the opportunity for activity and entertainment, and reflects positive aspects of urban life rather than the isolation and anonymity that is often seen to be the case.

(3) *Alienation and isolation.*
This factor contained items such as: apathy, dirty surroundings, loneliness, distrust, confusion, and violence. This factor predominantly includes items referring to characteristics of people but it also refers to the physical condition of the environment which is seen as something which fosters, or is a result of, a breakdown in interpersonal solidarity.

(4) *Good life.*
This factor contains items such as: intellectual people, affluent people, liberal people, prestigious place, old ways valued, and people who are interesting because they are not locals. This factor again refers to characteristics of the people but is elitist. Included here is the recognition of spatial mobility and innovation.

(5) *Privacy.*
This factor includes items such as: gossip, intrusion, ignorance and pettiness. This factor refers to a dimension of life involving privacy and carries a strong negative connotation with the inclusion of items noting pettiness and ignorance on the part of people.

(6) *Uncaring.*
This factor includes items such as: snobby people, depressing environment, and insensitive people. This factor represents the uncaring aspects of social climate and includes aspects of people's behaviour and feelings about the overall social life.

By using the above criteria it is possible to gain an impressionistic and subjective view of what it is like to live in a particular area. Such data may be collected informally by street interviews, for example, or by more formal techniques such as a social survey using a prepared question- naire. Many types of data will be included in a community assessment and may be influenced by the values and social goals of those involved in the writing of any report. While the distinctions between various sorts of data are not completely satisfactory it is often this subjective data which is missing.

This subjective data also gives us an indication of the availability of community ties and support structures which would be important if we wanted to utilize or mobilize community concern. It is also useful if we undertake the task of planning health care activities. For example, if we want to set up various evening groups it would be important to know if people felt it unsafe to be out at night. Attempts to offer new services or change existing provision without exploring the subjective views of residents may be unsuccessful.

In their study of self-help in an inner city, Knight and Hayes (1981) found that the social climate placed limits on the likelihood of small groups emerging and operating successfully. They conclude that postwar city planning was geared to solving physical problems rather than interpersonal or communal problems and that the opportunities to involve local people are being wasted in part because of the anomie and alienation which exist in inner city areas. In general, the lack of awareness of the concept of social climate has meant that little emphasis is given to ameliorating undesirable social conditions because it has not been thought possible to identify these in a measurable way.

Objective data

In order to measure conditions within a community there is a wide use of indicators to determine the social and health status. Health indicators include mortality and morbidity rates and there is only a limited degree of consensus on their use. It is more difficult to identify factors which reflect the social and economic aspects of an area which will inform us about the existence of deprivation or social need.

There is a lack of knowledge about what constitutes a social indicator. One cannot say with any certainty that any one factor is definitely an indicator of poor health or social problems.

IMPORTANT SOCIAL INDICATORS

Two of the key concepts in the social indicator literature are those of societal health (or the related notion of quality of life) and social currency (or the notion of a basic unit for social accounting such as time expenditure). It would be possible to assess the health of society in much the same way as we assess the health of the economy if there was agreement on key social goals and an indicator whose values are known which could be used when the goals had been achieved. This is difficult, however, and any effort to model social indicators is likely to incur considerable specification bias as one can never be certain that the effects observed are operative ones.

There is no way of ruling out the possibility that the effects are 'washed out' by causal forces not included in the analysis. Theories of society and social organization could be said to be more about concepts than variables. They are informed by things which have yet to be measured satisfactorily such as alienation and legitimacy. Connections between the theory of society and social statistics is not clear but this should not stop us trying to examine health status.

In social policy there has been a growing movement since the 1950s to use social indicators to identify groups or areas in need of social and health services and to subsequently develop programmes for the alleviation of deprivation. Any such programme must be one of positive action involving the allocation of additional resources on a partial basis. Problems arise, however, in the definition of social indicators for these types of programmes since they are concerned with complex levels of measurements involving large scale social programmes and social accounting such as that found in the analysis of unemployment figures. There are also implications here for social policy: not only does the application of positive discrimination assume a concentration of deprivation but it also assumes that such areas can be identified by means of social indicators. Within social policy this has been widely used in the field of education and housing. Social indicators for the identification of priority areas have been linked to specific programmes such as the Educational Priority Area Programme (known as EPA) and the Urban Programmes, General Improvement Areas and Housing Action Area Programmes.

These represent a further refinement of the concept in that the areas chosen are much smaller than local authorities and have as their underlying assumption the belief that these areas contain concentrated populations who suffer acute and multiple environmental and cultural handicaps. The Plowden Report (HMSO, 1967), from which emanated the Educational Priority Areas Programme, was the first statement prescribing the application of the positive discrimination principle in the social services field. A year later the Urban Programme (HMSO, 1986) was aimed at 'areas of acute need and included reference to the idea of localized districts which bear the marks of multiple deprivation'.

Health visiting and social indicators

Social indicators such as those described above are beginning to be used in health visiting. To date, however, the ratio of health visitors to population is not based on such indicators as social class, for example, which is shown to be related to health (Black Report, DHSS, 1980). Some health visitors produce an annual or bi-annual review of the caseload which is intended to identify characteristics that predict differential workload - even if prevalence rates, such as breastfeeding up to six weeks or smoking parents of under-one-year-old infants, are not yet included. It is particularly difficult to identify service strategies since these vary according to local population characteristics.

Although health visitor students undertake a community study which attempts to identify need based on a wide range of indicators, they are nevertheless given workloads based on institutional convenience such as general practitioners' caseloads. Little emphasis seems to be placed on matching need and resources. Perhaps this is because social indicators are not used or acknowledged as a valid way of determining health visiting priorities, or - again perhaps - this is due to the complex nature of determining what constitutes a social indicator.

Social indicators - definitions

Social indicators are constructs used to assess the current state of, and to measure changes in, socio-economic conditions of life in contemporary society (Land & McMillan, 1978). In 1967 the United States Department of Health Education and Welfare (US DHEW 1969) saw social indicators as the way forward for allocating resources. They described a social indicator as a statistic of direct normative interest which facilitates concise, comprehensive and balanced judgments about the major aspects of society. Since the issuing of this essentially simplistic statement there has been a growing body of literature which has exposed the very complex nature of using social indicators and the problems of classifying indicators in order to validate their use.

Hodge and Korman (1979) bring together the major themes which run through some of this literature, in that social indicators should be thought of as follows:

(1)   Should be differentiated in some meaningful way from economic ones.
(2)   Should reflect the achievement of national goals.
(3)   Ought to include their causes.
(4)   Should reveal the aggregate state of social well-being.
(5)   Should monitor social change.
(6)   Should reflect matters subject to manipulation by policy.

Four types of social indicators have been identified (Carlisle, 1972), as follows:

(1)   *Informative indicators:* these describe some part of the social system such as housing or education.
(2)   *Predictive indicators:* these enable extrapolations to be made from past and present measurements, e.g. economic activity.
(3)   *Problem-orientated indicators:* these are measures of social problem areas which may inform policy, e.g. crime rates.
(4)   *Programme evaluation indicators:* these are used as measurements of particular programmes, e.g. immunization rates.

In the UK, little use has been made of the last three types of indicators partly because policies tend to act to alter situations rather than solve problems. Edwards (1975) suggests that we make the most of a fifth type of social indicator which he calls a 'decision-making indicator' or low-level instrument to help facilitate the making of necessary decisions. Edwards defines this type of indicator as a variable, descriptive of certain demographic, environmental, pathological or service provision characteristics which are frequently aggregated on a geographical basis. These can be used alone or in conjunction with other variables to identify areas or aggregators of population with particular characteristics deemed relevant for the implementation of a social programme. Examples of this would be identification of inner city malaise.

The Black Report (DHSS 1980) also suggests that this type of social indicator has a use. Moreover, while the Standard Mortality Rate is the single best readily available indicator of need, it is insufficient on its own and other factors such as population characteristics and physical and environmental conditions need to be considered. The report acknowledges that social conditions not only are reflected in the infant mortality rate but are also important for the increased care needed among the survivors. It suggests that the proposals made by the Regional Allocation Working Party for weighting populations for community health services by age structure should be implemented. In addition, it is necessary to weight the number of children aged 0-4 for overcrowding, for family composition, for occupational class, and for unemployment. The difficulty of using social indicators for health planning is also highlighted. They state that the indicators of area deprivation available from the census provide a better tool for positive discrimination in housing policy than does health. There is a need for more relevant indicators which would enable the distribution of health care to be made on a more equitable basis.

The work of Chen *et al.* (1975) outlines the following important issues in determining social indicators for health:

(1)   The indicator should be of direct normative interest. This requires an implicit or explicit value component so that if the indicator improves, society can be considered better off.
(2)   The weighted index should be useful for priority setting, planning and evaluative research. This means that not only the direction but also the magnitude of the change in the indicator value is meaningful.
(3)   The indicator should be sufficiently sensitive to detect most of the important changes in health status – the mortality rate is no longer adequate as an indicator of health.
(4)   A community-wide health indicator should consist of clearly defined component parts and each part should make an independent contribution to what is studied
(5)   The indicator should be derived from observable data and be capable of being easily reproduced.

Thunhurst (1985) sets out three types of indicators which reflect deprivation:

(1)   Firstly, there are *direct indicators*. These consist of deprivations in themselves. Examples of these are severe overcrowding, single parent families, unemployment variables and variables concerned with social class.
(2)   Secondly, there are *indirect indicators*. These enable the existence of deprivation to be inferred, but do not necessarily constitute deprivations in themselves. Such variations are: households without a car; large households; numbers of children and pensioners. These variables can crudely be viewed as either proxy measures of possible lack of income, factors which might make poor households poorer, or measures of people likely to be discriminated against (e.g. those from the New Commonwealth or Asian subcontinent).

(3)   Thirdly, there are *interpretative indicators*. These are not mea-
       sures of deprivation, but aid the geographical analysis of the
       distribution of direct and indirect indicators. These include: the
       number of immigrants during the previous year; the number of
       council rented houses; the number of students; the amount of
       furnished and unfurnished rented accommodation.

Value judgments and social indicators

Social indicators and their relationship with social programmes are
neither objective nor value-free. By stressing the technical and statistical
aspects a veneer of objectivity and value freedom is placed on what is a
potentially politically divisive issue. Thus, by including certain indices
such as crime rates, delinquency or referral to social welfare services, it
is implied that deprivation has something to do with personal handicap
or inadequacy. To use data related to health and social service provision
is not to measure deprivation, or even need, but reflects present levels of
provision and departmental priorities (Smith & Jackson, 1988).

There is a tendency for those involved in social welfare studies to lump
together any variable that is vaguely relevant to social stress, disadvantage, social need, social pathology or social malaise and produce
composite indices of urban deprivation. This has diverted attention from
the need to clearly define deprivation. It has also delayed the recognition
that social indicators and social programmes are neither objective nor
value-free.

In using measures of social pathology attention is diverted from the
true nature of urban deprivation which results from social structure and
processes. As an example, urban deprivation can be seen as the
structural inability of some to compete in the markets which affect
people's life chances, such as employment, education and housing, and
which are interrelated. In other words, people may be bound together in
a complex set of relationships, and as an example it is possible that the
range of employment opportunities may be related to the type of
housing, educational opportunities and the area in which people live.

Hatch and Sherratt (1973) use two categories of variables, direct and
indirect indicators. The former are seen as constituting deprivations in
themselves whereas the latter may enable the inference that deprivations may be present but not constitute deprivations. Examples of direct
indicators are proportions of unfit housing or the proportion of children
receiving free school meals. Examples of indirect indicators are the
proportion of males in unskilled manual jobs or the proportion of large
households. The authors highlight the difficulty of drawing a firm line

between the two indicators and examine two sets of problems in identifying deprived areas, one theoretical and the other practical and empirical.

The theoretical problem is concerned with determining the causes of social deprivation and the reasons why deprivations are concentrated. The practical problem is to find indicators that are variable and have a clear and reliable relationship with the underlying deprivations they are supposed to indicate. In considering the relationship between the indicator and the underlying deprivation one is addressing the theoretical issue of causation.

Deprivation exists if the social norms expressed explicitly or implicitly in existing social policies are not attained. Norms about housing standards, for example, are implicit in a policy of providing improvement grants. In some cases, individual deprivations can be translated into area deprivation by aggregating them, e.g. the number of homes without a bath. Hatch and Sherratt suggest there are two types of deprived areas, one which is characterized by low social class and the other by the presence of immigrants and a mobile population. In their studies, it was found that deprivations in themselves were concentrated only to a limited extent and that any index that attempts to summarize a wide range of deprivations will neither be very efficient nor precise in identifying areas.

Deprivations seem to be widely, although unevenly, distributed in the inner city working-class areas. However, it must be said that areas suffering from multiple deprivation do not seem to form a separate category easily distinguished from other less deprived areas. In other words some people are not deprived because of the area in which they live, but rather they live in those areas because they are disadvantaged in housing, employment, health and education. This highlights the fact that urban deprivation has never been adequately defined. It is an ambiguous term and its nature and manifestations are constantly shifting. Urban deprivation according to Edwards (1975) is 'a description of the human condition and it is difficult to justify the moral qualification to measure fine degrees of misery. Any attempt at accuracy in the "arithmetic of woe" is spurious'. Social indicators will serve as one of a number of inputs to the decision-making process. They will be weighed against convenience, political expediency and notion of balance and fairness.

Edwards found that the use of area aggregated data about the characteristics of a population can be subject to misinterpretation. To the extent that the population of an area exhibit certain characteristics, for example, low income, unemployment, one-parent families, it is likely that they have brought that characteristic to the area and their concentration is a result of the ecological processes of social spacing effected largely through the operation of the housing market. Further, area social indicators do not indicate deprivation in an area but rather reflect the results of the operation of urban markets on people who are less qualified to compete in those markets. While recognizing these theoretical problems, some of the approaches which have been used in determining deprivation will be examined below.

Determining deprivation: some examples

A most useful source of statistical information about the relative social, economic and environmental deprivation of different towns and cities in England has been published from the census information (Department of the Environment 1981). (The 1991 census data will be available in 1992.) The idea behind the concept of multiple deprivation is that areas can fall into a cycle of decline because of a combination of problems such as high unemployment, overcrowded housing, high number of single parents or pensioners living alone, and a large exodus of the population. Any one or two of these factors might not cause alarm, indeed one can identify areas such as Hove and Eastbourne which despite having a high number of retired people living alone, are not areas of urban deprivation. It is the combination of problems associated with decline which have been analysed from the 1981 Census by the Department of Inner Cities Directorate. Government statisticians firstly identify eight indicators of deprivation for which figures were available. These were percentages in each local authority area for unemployment, overcrowded households, households lacking exclusive use of basic amenities, pensioners living alone, population change, mortality rate and households whose head was born either in the New Commonwealth or Pakistan.

The statisticians then identified which authorities fell in the worst ten and the worst 50 on each count. The results were as follows:

- The Isles of Scilly had the worst mortality rate
- Corby had the worst unemployment
- Tower Hamlets had the worst overcrowding
- Brent had the highest immigrant ranking
- Kensington had the highest population loss
- Hackney came in the worst ten nationally on as many as five out of the eight categories.

This analysis was then applied to the 80000 census enumeration districts, each made up of about 175 households, in order to ascertain how far each enumeration district is above or below the average for each characteristic. From this data a single index of deprivation was reached. While this may seem administratively neat there are problems in policy terms. Statistics for multiple deprivation appear to be less than straightforward and decision-makers seem to balance the facts with political judgments. Preston, for example, which has a higher deprivation score (on almost every system of measurement) than Rochdale, will not be awarded programme area status because there is a new town to help its development.

Many of the traditional deprivation blackspots which were awarded special status when the urban programme started in 1978, are now little worse than the national average. This is not because areas such as Gateshead or South Tyneside have improved but because the national average has worsened. Indeed, London boroughs take the top three places for overcrowding, numbers of single parents, lack of amenities, ethnic composition and population loss.

A study undertaken in Belfast (Belfast Areas of Special Social Needs 1976) demonstrated a close association between a series of indicators of economic and social disadvantage in defined areas of the city. The study used 20 indicators of social need to measure generally accepted aspects of disadvantage and 19 social characteristics which were interrelated with aspects of social need. Four main components of social need were identified:

(1) Unemployment – low family income
(2) Substandard housing – poor physical environment
(3) Personal handicap
(4) Educational disadvantage.

The study concluded that social need was concentrated in certain electoral wards which had high levels of many indicators of social deprivation. This approach, while identifying pockets of multiple deprivation, is not able to identify individuals outside these areas who might also be disadvantaged.

The application of positive discrimination policies on an area basis may therefore conflict with the needs of individuals. It may also conflict with territorial justice in that the relative needs of areas differ along a continuum with little demarcation between deprived and less deprived areas (Hatch & Sherratt, 1973).

In attempting to determine area indicators of social deprivation the Black Report suggests that the Census is a fruitful source of information. The Census provides information on a range of deprivation-related factors and is the principal source of ecological data on social conditions. Imber (1977) used Census indicators to classify areas in need of social services; since there is a close connection between the need for social services and preventive health care (Black Report DHSS 1980), Imber's work is therefore a useful focus for identifying indicators which may be used in assessing community health needs.

Imber lists ten variables and suggests that overcrowding has the highest correlation with all other indicators. In other words, if a family lives in overcrowded conditions there is a likelihood that some other indicators of need may be present:

  (1)   Overcrowding
  (2)   Private rented furnished accommodation
  (3)   Lack of amenities
  (4)   Lone pensioners
  (5)   Unemployed
  (6)   Social class V
  (7)   Working mothers
  (8)   One-parent family
  (9)   Large families
 (10)   Council housing.

From these indicators we can see that people who cannot compete in the job market, e.g. the unemployed, may therefore be unable to compete in the housing markets. While recognizing that much more work is needed on the relationships between indicators of social disadvantage and mortality the Black Report shows that the following indicators appear to reflect areas of deprivation:

(1)   Overcrowding
(2)   Unemployment
(3)   Unskilled workers
(4)   Families with four or more children
(5)   Perinatal mortality
(6)   Infant mortality
(7)   Adjusted mortality ratio (this is the local death rate standardized for population divided by the national rate).

Jarman (1983) has detailed the following social factors and service factors which contribute to the pressure of work on general practitioners.

Social factors

(1)   Older people (aged 65 and over)
(2)   Children (aged under 5)
(3)   Unemployment
(4)   Poor housing
(5)   Ethnic minorities (people born outside the UK)
(6)   Single-parent households
(7)   Elderly living alone
(8)   Overcrowding
(9)   Lower social class
(10) Highly mobile people (percentage changing house in a year)
(11) Non-married couple families (less stable family groups)
(12) Difficulties visiting (long distances, traffic, etc.).

Service factors

(1)   Long outpatient waiting times
(2)   Low percentage of area health authority expenditure on community services, more on hospital services
(3)   Low percentage of local authority expenditure on home helps, meals on wheels
(4)   Low percentage of area health authority nurses attached to general practices
(5)   High percentage of elderly GPs (aged 70+) in area
(6)   High percentage of single-handed GPs in area
(7)   High percentage of GPs' lists over 3000
(8)   High percentage of GPs' lists under 1000.

Simply to compile a list of indicators is of limited use, as many categories of indicators overlap or are mutually exclusive. It may be more useful to examine combinations of indicators. It is of limited use to know the number of one-parent families in an area, but to know how many of these families live in privately rented accommodation lacking basic amenities may be more useful.

The identification and application of social indicators is a complex exercise and their usage is fraught with the difficulties outlined. There would appear to be some consensus however that certain indicators are related to deprivation, and social need and therefore might be used in determining the health of the community.

CONCLUSION

This chapter provides an overview of the developments in primary health care and community health at national and international level. Considerable emphasis has been placed on the determining of social indicators as this is an important issue in identifying health needs. The changes in health and social policies mean that health visitors and other community health workers must be involved in this aspect of planning. They have unique access to a wide range of the population and are able to contribute not only to the most traditional indices of health, but also to the more subjective data which is often missing from the official figures, but which is crucial to the lives and health of the community.

Events associated with these key health areas should be an integral part of the family health assessment and family record. In this way, community-based strategies can be linked to need.

3 Health Visiting and the Community

Jean Orr

WORKING AT A COMMUNITY LEVEL

Health visitors have a considerable contribution to make in the arena of community health and many are actively involved in this area. There needs to be more examination of the issues surrounding the role of the nurse in the community, the compilation of community health profiles, the encouragement of participation, and the formulation of new strategies of intervention.

Health visitors should be able to assist communities to recognize and meet their collective needs (Goeppinger *et al.*, 1982) by identifying problems and assets in the community and intervening to strengthen the interactions within the community. This approach can be described as working with the constituent parts of that unit, i.e. with individuals and families. It is a common assumption to equate delivering health visiting to individuals and families who happen to live in the community, with working as a health visitor concerned with community health issues. However, operating at a community level means working with various groups and networks, not concentrating only on individuals and families. It is a move away from 'the card equals the client syndrome'. This wider community involvement also means being involved in community development which is seen as bringing about change by consensus and may even mean community action which seeks to bring change by conflict. It means urging demands on local or central government and on professionals for innovations or change in the pattern of health provision and the allocation of resources. There are considerable problems and tensions within the area of community health and it may be that there are no local solutions to problems of inequality and economic policies. Often community health workers feel most comfortable addressing marginal issues such as local playgroup provision, but see no role in the wider issue of the economic policies which affect children.

There are particular assumptions which underpin working at a community level, irrespective of the type of worker involved. Some of these assumptions are detailed by the Community Projects Foundation

(1982) and need consideration by health visitors. Community work is said to be based on the belief that people have the capacity to join together and take action on their own behalf. The role of the worker is to stimulate this capacity even in severely deprived areas. The underlying assumption is that the provision of services is more likely to be taken up if they are geared to the needs and priorities which have been articulated by the local people. It is imperative for the worker to get to know the community from the inside in order to help members formulate needs and priorities from which to facilitate self-help activities and negotiate with relevant authorities. The aim is to develop skills of collective activity, help decision-making processes and facilitate the residents to manage their own institutions (Henderson & Thomas, 1980). Community work engages groups rather than individuals and it aims to change the environment rather than adapt people to it. Essentially, community work attempts to build on strengths, rather than identify weakness. The number and range of community health initiatives are growing and there is now a well defined community health movement in Britain (Rosenthal, 1983). This movement is characterized by being:

(1)   Based outside the health professionals.
(2)   Concerned with inequalities in health and health care provision.
(3)   Based on the belief that the achievement of a healthy community depends on a collective awareness of the social causes of ill-health and positive health.
(4)   Challenging, at an individual and collective level, the monopoly of information about health and ill-health by health professionals.

In recent years there has been a rapid growth of community health initiatives throughout the country. This would suggest that somehow statutory services have failed to meet the needs of clients. As Drennan (1986) suggests:

 'The very point the community health projects are making is that people should be able to gain access to knowledge and information in an appropriate way and gain confidence in using it – that will only happen when health professionals like health visitors are openly able to share their knowledge and expertise and engage in an equitable dialogue with the communities they work in.'

The organizational setting for any professional presents problems if that organization is bureaucratic in nature. This is because the authority in a bureaucracy is structural, while professional authority is more charismatic. Etzioni (1964) sees a conflict between the enforced and sanctioned values of the former and the internalized values of the latter. The conflict may be most evident in the area of service delivery. Policy makers often fix on one method as a panacea to service delivery problems and prematurely foreclose options on other methods. While this may achieve bureaucratic goals it may not be in the best interests of the professional goals, in this case, health visiting.

For health visitors to operate at a community level they have to recognize themselves in both leadership and change agent role. But how ready are health visitors and their managers to develop leadership and change potential?

Blattner (1981) suggests the following self-assessment questions, first to evaluate leadership potential, and second to assess your motivation as a change agent.

'Do you see yourself as an activist?'

(1) Do you recognize the possibility of change?
(2) Do you believe in a particular project or plan?
(3) Are you willing to invest in a few hours to gather some data and to do some critical thinking?
(4) Are you willing to help bring a few other interested colleagues and residents together to formulate a plan or project?
(5) Do you enjoy eliciting information, suggestions, and ideas from people?
(6) Can you patiently allow others to arrive at decisions at their own pace?
(7) Can you keep a sense of humour when under pressure?
(8) Do you get defensive when attacked?
(9) Can you educate people without preaching to them?
(10) Can you avoid taking sides and remain impartial and objective in a situation that requires it?

'Do you see yourself as a change agent?'

(1) Does your motivation stem from a genuine desire to improve something?
(2) Does your motivation stem from a personal desire for power or recognition?
(3) Do you want to change simply for change's sake or to keep things from stagnating?

(4) Does the situation call for interpersonal or highly developed organizational skills? Do you have them?
(5) How much experience have you had with this particular type of problem?
(6) What are your credentials? Are you regarded as an expert according to the key people in your situation?
(7) Is your personality suited to the particular situation?

Drennan (1986) identified several issues as being essential to the development of the health visitor's role in community work; however, this would also apply to other community health nurses.

- A clear understanding of and a commitment to this method of work.
- A support mechanism to provide support, guidance and monitoring of work.
- A knowledge of participation in informal group settings.
- Time to prepare and conduct work (this has implications for policy making. It requires commitment from the employers, authority for allocation of services, flexibility of working hours).
- Good working relationships with health education departments.
- The need for continuing evaluation.

Some health visitors see themselves as fulfilling these roles and one of the unique features of health visiting has been its ability to adapt and respond to local needs and changing perspectives. In addition, there is evidence that some health visitors are being both creative and innovatory in practice (Dowling, 1983; Orr, 1982). At a conference on 'Community Dimensions in Health: Addressing the Confusions' held at the King's Fund Centre in London in June 1984, many health visitors described new approaches, some of which are outlined below.

Examples of a new approach

The Rochdale Family Service Unit's Young Parents' Project is a specialized service for young families. It concentrates on developing practical skills through group work, breaking down isolation through self-help support, and follow-up by home visiting and befriending the families at home (Courtney, 1984).

Work with a wide variety of community groups to raise health and health services awareness has been described by Drennan (1984). These groups ranged from immigrant workers to groups in unemployment centres, youth and pensioner groups.

A study by Drennan (1986) of 130 district health authorities showed that health visitors are involved in a wide range of community initiatives. These fall into eight categories:

- Health campaigns and health screening schemes.
- The formation of, or representation on, special interest or pressure groups. These covered a wide range of groups, e.g. tenants' associations, sickle cell society and under-five resource centre.
- Provision of health information at local events such as agricultural shows.
- Collaborating with other workers to produce information resources.
- Involvement in health education in the workplace.
- Use of local media for discussion of health topics.
- Taking part in community development initiatives such as unemployed groups, rape crisis centres, neighbourhood health projects

The overall conclusion of this study is that although some health visitors do become involved in community activities constraints are imposed by large caseloads, lack of management support, and scarcity of accommodation and funding. It emerges that health visitors work with a wide range of clients; they also come under pressure from policy-makers to get more involved with older people.

In Brent, the Chalkhill Neighbourhood Project has a multidisciplinary team of social workers, community workers, health visitors and an administrator based in a flat on the Chalkhill Estate. As members of this team, health visitors have moved away from their traditional role with individual families and have begun expanding the community development elements of their work. They have participated in initiating a youth advisory service, under-fives week, women's group, parenting group, mental health group, pilot scheme for the elderly confused, toy library and play group. An aim is to influence fieldworkers and managers within the statutory services to adopt a community involvement and consultation approach (Dennis & Wickstead, 1984; Sachs, 1990).

Billingham's work in Nottingham is an excellent example of working with the community and in particular with women to improve health and uptake of services (Billingham, 1991). Drennan (1988), in her book on health visitors and groups, provides an analysis of ten innovative case studies of work with groups. These cover a wide range of situations including a tranquillizer support group, improving health care for the homeless, the Riverside Child Health Project, and community action.

Caseload or community

Health visitors have such widespread access to the families and individuals which make up any community that there is therefore considerable potential to develop this area of work. There are difficulties, however, in defining what the proper determinants of the health visitor's workload are and the relationship between the individual families visited and the wider community. The families obviously form part of the community, are influenced by it and in turn influence it; when a health visitor visits a family therefore she is conscious of the health impact of the surrounding community (Fig. 3.1).

Health visitors hold considerable information both about their own caseloads and the local community. This information is seldom collated. Indeed there is a debate within health visiting itself as to whether health visitors should be involved in compiling either a caseload profile or a community study. These are not alternative procedures, rather they are complementary and are used for different purposes. Each health visitor must, as a prerequisite, know her caseload in considerable detail before she can determine priorities and allocate resources. Two models of caseload analysis that have actually been used in practice are presented

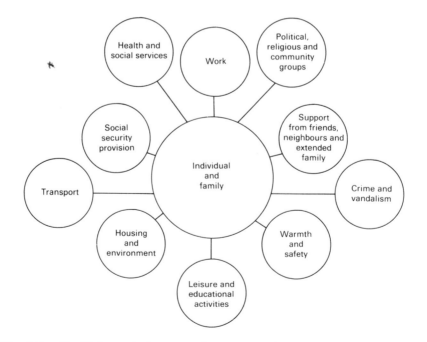

Fig. 3.1.   Health impact of surrounding community.

later (see Appendices 1 and 2). To determine the relationship between a caseload and a community health profile, we need to examine how case loads are determined.

Attached caseload

An attached caseload means that health visitors have a caseload that is based on a general practitioner's practice population. While this ought to mean the entire population registered with that general practitioner, in reality it means the families with children under five and some elderly people. Health visitors in this system should be able to undertake a detailed caseload analysis from which to identify a range of priorities. The problem is that the caseload will cut across many communities and networks.

There are fundamental problems associated with attachment in terms of access to records and it could be argued that health visitors have not hitherto had adequate access to general practice records. Where age/sex registers do exist it may be that these are not made available to nursing staff. Even if age/sex registers are available widespread dispersion of the practice population means that community initiatives such as group work cannot be undertaken and social and health indicators cannot be used to determine spatial disadvantage. In particular, it will be difficult to use databases such as the census. The practice population in reality does not act as a database even though this should be one of its main attractions. Computerized records should enable a detailed analysis of all people registered with the practice but what may not be recorded are the social and economic circumstances of the family: consideration of the health impact of society on families is fundamental in health visiting.

There is also a disparity between community care, with its emphasis on using families, social networks and community resources, and the reality of attachment to non-zoned general practice. Social networks, on which much of community care is based, are located spatially and it is difficult to see how health visitors can be aware of such networks and voluntary groups if they visit over a wide area. Not all families register with a general practitioner and this is especially true of those who might be most vulnerable.

Geographical caseload

With the geographical caseload system, health visitors have responsibility for a defined geographical area and at first glance this system may offer more possibility for community involvement. The problem is that the geographical area may not have any of the features normally associated with a community; indeed it may include many different communities. It is often the case that areas are divided on a very arbitrary basis: dividing a town into three parts, for example, or dividing a housing estate in two, thus diminishing the possibility of fully working with the community. Where health visitors have a geographical patch, however, they can identify local groups more easily than their attached colleagues. It may also be easier to keep contact with what Dowling (1983) calls 'invisible' families who do not register with general practitioners or become involved with any of the health services.

In some areas health visitors are now introducing corporate caseloads. In this system, the caseload is shared out between health visitors: thus families are not necessarily linked to one health visitor. In other areas, health visitors contract with clients. This involves the health visitor and client in drawing up a contract of visits. To date, neither of these approaches has been evaluated.

District Health Profile

As there is little uniformity in determining caseloads, it is difficult to see how one health visitor or community nurse can draw up a community health profile without using information from her colleagues and agreeing on a profile which will be relevant on a collective basis.

What is suggested is a mixture of two approaches – the caseload profile and the community profile – which would provide opportunities for working with groups in need, spatially, and on a client basis. This would result in the compilation of a District Health Profile (Fig. 3.2).

Health visiting/community nurse caseload profile	Community health profile
Based on existing records	Context of socio/economic health indicators
Related to individuals and families	Identifies at-risk groups
	Identifies resources
Not spatially focussed	Recognizes discrete communities/is spatially focussed
Includes many communities	
	Includes the perceptions of local residents

Fig. 3.2.   District Health Profile.

However, it should be emphasized that a community profile is different from a caseload analysis and operates at a different level of abstraction and analysis. By examining the difference between neighbourhood and community, we will now present an operational definition of community and suggest how a community profile might be undertaken.

This lack of conceptual clarity encourages students and health visitors to use the terms neighbourhood and community interchangeably. However, from what has been explored in the previous chapter about the nature of community, this approach negates any ideas of a community of interests and focuses mainly on the spatial aspects of shared locality.

Entanglement of the study of communities with the study of neighbourhoods creates a number of problems, including the following:

(1) The identification of a neighbourhood as a focus for communal ties assumes a belief in spatial determinism, i.e. the organizing power of space. Although it may be likely that space-time costs encourage some local relationships it does not follow that there is a strong degree of social organization in the neighbourhood.

(2) The presence of many local relationships does not necessarily create discrete neighbourhoods. There may be overlapping ties affected by individual needs and physical mobility.

(3) The concentration on local ties omits other major sets of relationships, which operate outside neighbourhoods. Work relationships are an example of this omission.

(4) To focus on the neighbourhood may give undue importance to spatial characteristics as the determinant of social behaviour, e.g. vandalism.

(5) Many of the neighbourhood studies concentrate on the existence of locally organized behaviour and sentiments and when these are not observed it is often assumed by students that the community has decayed or does not exist.

(6) The traditional concept of neighbourhood has less meaning than the micro-neighbourhood as represented by small groupings of houses or one or two blocks of flats (Marans, 1976).

An examination of the urban sociological literature shows that there are a number of reasons why the concept of neighbourhood has been substituted for that of community (Wellman & Leighton, 1979).

(1) The neighbourhood is an easily identifiable unit and therefore useful for researching small-scale interactions.

(2) Some researchers have seen the neighbourhood as a microcosm of

the city and the city as a collection of neighbourhoods, thus missing the importance of large scale urban structures.
(3) Planners have identified spatial areas and treated these as coherent neighbourhoods and have seen these as some type of natural phenomenon.
(4) The emphasis on spatial distributions has led to the mistaken view that territory is the most important organizing factor in urban social relations.
(5) There has been a concern with studying conditions which maintain solidarity sentiments and the neighbourhood has been studied as an apparent focus of normative solidarity.

The concentration on neighbourhood has had a strong impact on definitions of, research on, and theorizing about the concept of community. This concentration has produced considerable evidence about how small-scale social systems operate in a variety of social contexts. But does the concept of neighbourhood equate with the concept of community? Wellman and Leighton (1979) would say it does not. Definitions of community tend to include three ingredients, as follows:

(1) Networks of interpersonal ties which provide sociability and support to members.
(2) Residence in a common locality.
(3) Solidarity sentiments and activities.

It is principally the emphasis on common locality, and to a lesser extent the emphasis on solidarity, which has encouraged the identification of community with neighbourhood. It could be argued, however, that spatial distribution variables are mainly important in as much as they effect the formations of interpersonal networks and the flow of resources through such networks.

In the context of health visiting, we need to be concerned with neighbourhoods and communities. People tend to have strong ties with both neighbourhood and community and receive support from a number of relationships. An individual's primary network will most probably include neighbourhood relationships but will also include a variety of ties with distant relatives, workmates, close friends, and so on, resulting in a widespread and flexible network of relationships. Health visitors, therefore, need to consider a more 'operational' definition of community.

Operational definition of community

While recognizing the complexities of defining community (discussed in

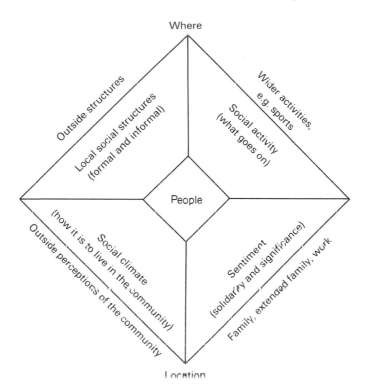

Fig. 3.3. Operational definition of community.

Chapter 2), it may be useful to present an operational definition identifying the major components of community and explore what these mean for health visiting (Fig. 3.3). These various components are important for the health visitor if she wants to undertake any community initiatives. For example, if a health visitor wants to initiate a meeting to explore the interest in a well women's clinic, she will need to consider these aspects (Fig. 3.4).

THE ROLE OF THE HEALTH VISITOR WITHIN THE COMMUNITY

The health visitor's role within communities may vary according to local situations but it is possible to suggest the following broad functions:

(1) To compile a community health profile and keep this updated.
(2) To identify priorities with residents and mobilize resources.

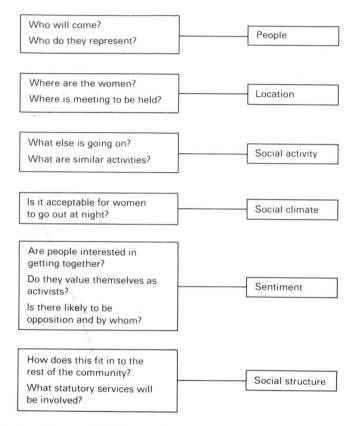

Fig. 3.4. Application of definition of community.

(3) To organize groups to effect increase in knowledge of health affecting practices.
(4) To act as a link between local people and the health services and to facilitate a two-way flow of information.
(5) To provide an outreach programme.
(6) To act as a catalyst for change.

   Health visitors need to compile a community profile as the first major step preceding intervention in community issues. This work will involve assembling knowledge about the community that will inform decisions about health policy and practice. There is, however, some concern about the ethics of collecting information about a community both from statutory and informal sources. Health visitors are usually concerned about the indiscriminate and unreported collecting of information, but even though we may accept this to be for the general good of society, it could also be seen as an invasion of privacy. Who gives health visitors the mandate to collect information and make judgments about a locality and its people? This is particularly pertinent when we recognize that the people themselves may have no intention of utilizing our services.

Pinker (1982) draws attention to the issues of information gathering in his critique of the community model of social work. This model, he says, would mean 'a proliferation of local databanks based largely on hearsay, gossip and well-meaning but uninvited prying'. Additionally, the development of preventive social work on a local base would threaten the right to privacy in that it would mean enquiries being made into the personal circumstances of citizens. There are problems in determining a balance between the desire to locate and provide for unexpressed needs and the rights of citizens to maintain their privacy. This is an issue which health visitors must confront before further developing a community based model of practice.

Fruin (1971) highlights some other issue in data collection. he considers that data should be:

(1) *Collectable.* It is pointless attempting to collect data which the interviewer is afraid or embarrassed to ask.
(2) *Correct.* It may be that some case files are low on reliability.
(3) *Complete.* Incomplete coverage may prove useless.
(4) *Comparable.* Much potential value is lost if there is no means to compare with other areas or groups. In addition, data collection needs to be consistent for comparability over time.
(5) *Concise.* Too much data may lead to confusion.

THE COMMUNITY HEALTH PROFILE

The compilation of a Community Health Profile will involve the health visitor in examining the following 12 topics and drawing on knowledge from sociology, psychology, epidemiology and social policy.

(1) Historical, environmental and spatial characteristics
(2) Organizations
(3) Residents
(4) Social climate
(5) Social and economic features
(6) Power and leadership
(7) Health status

(8)   Social services
(9)   Health services
(10) Health visiting services
(11) Health action potential
(12) Health needs assessment, action and evaluation.

When these 12 topics are considered separately, the following break-down emerges:

Historical, environmental and spatial characteristics

- History
- Location boundaries and geographical features
- General environment
- Housing
- Transport networks
- Facilities, e.g. shops, post offices
- Industries

Organizations

- Local and central government
- Religious groups
- Voluntary groups
- Community groups
- Self-help groups
- Political groups

Residents

- Social class distribution
- Age/sex structure
- Values and traditions
- Family living patterns, standards and routines
- Existence of vulnerable groups, e.g. gypsy families
- Personal handicap
- Ethnic minorities

Social climate: residents' perceptions

- Warmth and closeness
- Activity and entertainment

- Alienation and isolation
- Good life
- Privacy
- Uncaring

Social and economic features

- Employment
- Educational facilities and attitudes
- Recreation facilities
- Household composition
- Level of overcrowing
- Population movement
- Crime and vandalism
- Number receiving social security benefits

Power and leadership

- Business and organized labour
- Elective politics
- Administrative politics
- Community politics

Health status

- Mortality and morbidity rates for all age groups
- Accident rates by social class and age groups
- Health risks, e.g. pollution
- Stress factors, e.g. poverty
- Health problems, e.g. drug misuse
- Use of services
- Suicide rates
- Number of children on 'at risk' registers of Health and Social Services

Social services

- Provision of statutory social services
- Liaison with health services
- Shortfalls
- Voluntary social services groups in particular self-help groups
- Provision of residential accommodation

Health services

- Hospital services
- Community health services
- Shortfalls
- Liaison in services
- Management structure of services
- Community Health Councils

Health visiting services

- Location and setting
- Caseload analysis
- Liaison with other workers/groups
- Range of duties
- Constraints
- Use of services

Health action potential

- Resources such as friends, families and networks
- Sources of help outside recognized agencies
- Amount of changes the community has achieved in other areas
- The relationship of health and education to other community concerns
- Community's openness to change

Health needs assessment and proposed action and evaluation

- National level
- District level
- Professional level
- Community level

Compiling a community health profile

In order to compile a community health profile the health visitor will be involved in the following:

(1) Obtaining the feel of the area and gaining the residents' perceptions of the need.
(2) Examining local sources of data.
(3) Examining national sources of data.

As a first step in becoming acquainted with the area the health visitor will need to spend time looking around and talking to local people in informal settings. Time will need to be spent in the streets visiting shops and cafés and local amenities on different days and at different times. During this period the health visitor will be observing the general appearance of the area and attempting to determine the general pattern of life.

A guide to the type of features that might be observed is given below:

Environment

- Is it a well kept area?
- Is there litter and broken glass around?
- Is there much graffiti?
- Where are the schools?
- Are there play spaces?
- What transport services exist?
- What amenities are there, e g parks?
- Are there local shops; are they expensive?
- Where are the major employment centres?

Housing

- What type of housing exists?
- Is it well kept?
- Is it near shops and other amenities?
- What are prices in estate agents?
- What houses/flats are advertised in local shops?

What would it be like for me to live here?

- Is it very different from my community?
- What leisure facilities would I use?
- Are there convenient buses and trains?
- Would I be pleased to live here?
- What would I like and dislike about the area?
- What facilities exist for my family?
- Can I identify with the local people or are they different from me?

General features

- Are clinics, doctors, dentists, chemists situated near to housing?
- Who goes to the unemployment exchange or job centre?

- What is the queue like at the post office for child benefits and pensions?
- Are there many pubs – who uses them?
- Is there bingo – who goes?
- What kind of people are in the streets (e.g. young, old, male, female, and so on) and does this vary at night?
- Are there any groups hanging about street corners?
- Do people tend to chat to each other, e.g. in shops?
- Which community groups are advertised in local shops and clinics?

Useful information can be gained from studying local newspapers, free sheets and radio programmes. In particular, any local radio phone-in problem programme may pinpoint current issues. The existence of local self-help groups or a local campaign will often be highlighted in the letters page of the newspaper. The local library is a useful source of information on local activities.

Local people can also be interviewed informally about what it is like to live in the area. Such activity can be carried out in such settings as local clinics, shopping centres, libraries and community halls. What the health visitor is interested in is how it is for these people to be part of their community.

Throughout the community there are a range of people who have contact with a wide cross-section of local residents and who are a useful source of data. Examples of such groups of people include clergy, teachers, café owners, shopkeepers, the Citizens' Advice Bureau, publicans, play-group leaders and the Community Health Council. Other workers may be able to give information, e.g. youth workers, social security officers, Trade Union officials, social workers and the police.

There are also a number of individuals within areas who exercise influence through informal networks which exist throughout communities. These key people may be actively involved in local pressure groups or residents' committees or act more covertly by lobbying decision makers. It is necessary to understand that power within a community may not always reside in the elected representatives. In interviewing such key people it is necessary to know how long the individuals have been in the area, their participation in existing organizations, and to wehat extent they share the interests and values of the other residents. For example, if we were interviewing the local clergy then we might get a different view of an area from that given by a welfare rights worker. It is also necessary to recognize that individuals have their own prejudices and values and what is said has to be set against information obtained from other sources.

During this time it will be useful to interview local people in order to find out the issues deemed relevant by the residents and to attempt to determine the social climate. This was the approach adopted by Knight and Hayes (1981), who interviewed a small sample of local residents chosen at random from the electoral register. The problems perceived by their samples were classified into eight main types:

(1) Crime
(2) Other inhabitants
(3) Race
(4) Teenagers
(5) Poor facilities and services
(6) Decaying physical environment
(7) Population density
(8) Bad reputation of area

We can see that many of these issues are similar to those related to social climate and also include indicators related to social deprivation.

Learning about an area is an ongoing exercise and further information, when known, will be added to the database. However, it is important to form a first opinion from personal observation and interactions before looking at other sources of data and becoming 'contaminated' by official views. Essentially, it has to be recognized that information about any area is seldom value-free and reflects the problems we have highlighted in examining social indicators.

Local sources of data

Many of the local services publish information which will be useful to health visitors but this information may mainly reflect current service provision and should not be taken as a prior indicator to need.

Agencies which may be contacted to ascertain what is available about local conditions include the following:

(1) *Social Services Departments*, e.g. provision of home helps, children received into care.
(2) *Local Voluntary Services Agency.* They will be able to identify local voluntary groups and indicates studies undertaken by voluntary agencies, e.g. Age Concern.
(3) *Housing Department*, e.g. rent rebates, waiting lists, eviction orders, rent arrears.

(4) *Local Education Authority*, e.g. physically, mentally, aurally, and visually handicapped children of school age, referrals to child guidance, children in receipt of free school meals.

(5) *Police*, e.g. crime rates, type of crime, juvenile offenders.

(6) *Department of Social Security*, e.g. households in receipt of benefit, numbers in receipt of child benefit, family income supplements.

(7) *Department of Employment*, e.g. numbers of long-term employed, uptake of youth opportunity schemes.

(8) *District Health Authorities*. The collection of information regarding health statistics and health services utilization.

The collection of such information is a major responsibility of District Health Authorities and should provide a most valuable source of information for health visitors on such matters as clinic attendance and infant mortality. In the context of the North West of England, for example, a useful source of data is the comparative community health statistics published by the regional Statistical Unit of the North Western Regional Health Authority. In addition to routinely collected statistics there are studies undertaken at the request of management or by individuals pursuing research interests. Details of such studies should be available from the district management teams.

National sources of data

A major function of government is the collection of information and this provides the health visitor with considerable sources of data. Official statistics publications can be divided into three main types:

(1) Summary publications which bring together statistics from various departmental publications, e.g. Social Trends.

(2) Regular primary sources of statistics such as the General Household Survey and the Census.

(3) Occasional papers and commissioned reports such as the Court Report (DHSS, 1976b).

A comprehensive list of useful sources of information is given in Appendix 4; however, the following may be of particular value to health visitors:

(1) *Social Trends*. This is the main summary publication and presents a wide range of social statistics in an easily understood manner and

is published annually. Topics that are covered include population, employment, expenditure, health services, housing, education and the environment.

(2) *Abstract of Regional Statistics.* These abstracts are published annually and present a detailed quantitative picture of regional variations throughout the UK and across a broad range of topics, social, demographic and economic.

(3) *General Household Survey.* This survey provides data on personal expenditure and income, family composition, housing, employment, illness, medical attention, educational qualifications and personal social services.

(4) *Registrar General's Report.* These reports are weekly returns and quarterly returns, and they cover a range of vital statistics, e.g. mortality and morbidity rates.

(5) *Registrar General's Statistical Review.* This review is published annually in three parts: medical tables on deaths, etc., population tables on marriage, births, etc., commentaries on the trends and developments in the year.

Health visitors may complain that national sources such as the above are not particularly useful in determining local needs because of the size of the units examined. National sources do, however, allow comparisons to be made and the Census does provide one of the most useful sources of information.

What is the Census?

Every ten years the Government carries out a full Census in the United Kingdom to obtain information on which to base national, regional and local policies for planning, housing, education, employment and so on. In addition, five years after each full Census, there is a Sample Census of 10% of the population.

The country is divided up into enumeration districts (EDs). These are areas small enough to be covered by one Census enumerator on the Census Day and they usually contain between 50 and 200 households. The Census questionnaire is designed to gather information about the characteristics of the population, its housing and several other special topics, as follows:

(1) Information collected and published on the *population* of an area: total population; age and sex of the population; size of households;

number of employed and unemployed by age and sex; numbers and type of people in hospitals, hotels and other institutions; country of birth.

(2)   Information collected and published on *housing* in an area: details of size and type of housing; number of persons per room; amenities (e.g. bath, WC, hot and cold water supply) in the dwelling; the number of persons and households in different tenure groups (e.g. owner occupiers, tenants sharing dwellings and amenities); number of vacant dwellings.

(3)   More detailed information is available on *special topics* such as: types of people moving house and where they move to and from; the employment and class structure of the population; educational qualifications of the population.

Once obtained, the information is then summarized in tables relating to different sized areas from EDs (the smallest unit) to countries (England, Scotland and Wales). In between are: wards, parishes, local authority areas, new towns, conurbations, counties, sub-regions, regions, cities, boroughs and rural districts.

The Census information is published in three main forms:

(1)   *National Tables* – provide information on a wide range of subjects for areas ranging from rural districts to the whole country.

(2)   *County Reports* – produced for each county in Great Britain.

(3)   *Ward Library Tables or Small Area Statistics* – provide information on EDs, wards and parishes. These are published in three sheets for each ED, ward and parish:
       Sheet 1: called 100% Population. This gives figures on age, sex, birthplace, employment figures and residency in hospitals, etc.
       Sheet 2: called 100% Households. This gives figures on housing standards, tenancies, type of household – e.g. those with children; number of shared households.
       Sheet 3: called 10% Sample. This gives information on the number of people who have moved, type of jobs held by residents, e.g. women in full/part-time jobs and number of children in two-parent and one-parent families.

The County reports, published in three volumes, give figures for counties, local authority areas, new towns and conurbations, e.g. Greater Manchester. The first volume gives age, sex and country of birth, numbers employed and unemployed and the number of single and married people.

The second volume gives information on how households occupy dwellings, e.g. how many people occupy how many rooms. The third volume gives figures on housing, e.g. the amenities and the number of tenants and owner occupiers.

When reading Census publications there are a number of points to remember:

(1) Always read the explanatory notes and definitions.
(2) If the figures relate to the 10% sample of households you will have to add a '0' to all the figures in order to talk about all the population in the area.
(3) Census information may not be completely accurate. It is thought that inaccuracies occur most often in data relating to multi-occupation or sharing in housing.
(4) Data may become out of date because of the long time gap between censuses.
(5) Definitions of terms used may also change between censuses.
(6) Geographical boundaries may change between censuses.

The Census contains a considerable amount of information and the following are some examples of useful indicators:

(1) Children under 5
(2) School-age children
(3) Pensioners (males over 65, females over 60)
(4) One-parent families
(5) Number of unemployed – males and females by age
(6) Social class derivable from socio-economic group
(7) Hours of work of all women, married women and women with children under 5 (see Appendix 3 for further details).

The most recent Census was carried out in 1991 and much of the information is not yet available. Readers are advised to contact their local HMSO bookshop or the Office of Population Census and Surveys (OPCS) if they would like more information. Census information, as it becomes available, is accompanied by User Guides which are supplied by OPCS Customer Services.

The Regional/Health Authority and 'old' Health District constitutions are also available (User Guide 8). The unpublished Small Area Statistics (SAS) became available at the beginning of 1984. These were at the new District Health level (User Guides 81 and 52).

IDENTIFICATION OF HEALTH NEEDS WITHIN THE NHS REFORMS

Each Health Authority has to collect, collate and present health status information for policy making decisions at a local level. To contribute to this database, health visitors should develop strategies which demonstrate their own particular contribution to the aims of the Health Authority involved.

The specific contribution of the nurse or health visitor should now be recognized as feeding into this new policy making machinery with appropriate prevalence rates and information about the impact of the presence/absence of backup resources.

With the emphasis on making the best use of health visiting resources, there is much debate about the introduction of skill mix within the health visiting service. At present, there is little evidence as to how this is to be managed. Some management reinforces traditional and entrenched practices by opting for task analysis rather than any analysis of the level of decision making or the level of discretion expected. This has ramifications for the level of quality which can be achieved.

If Districts are to determine health needs, the rationing process must be more explicit as it is clear that not all needs can be met. The issue will centre on whose needs take priority. For example, the closure of family planning clinics is going against consumer choice but fits in with the shift of services to general practitioners. The process of identifying health needs has been described by Anderson *et al.* (1978) as:

(1) Defining the database
(2) Stating the problem
(3) Examining causative factors
(4) Determining short- and long-term objectives
(5) Initiating plans
(6) Measuring outcome against stated objectives.

A major criticism of health visitors is that they stop at identifying the health needs. Few proceed to analyse these needs, or to consider how they might be met and by whom. This may be as a result of a confusion about the first experience students have of undertaking a study of community health needs or it may be because of a reluctance to see health needs in the wider socio–political context (Fig. 3.5).

In order to identify specific groups within the community, health visitors could utilize the major social/health indicators discussed pre-

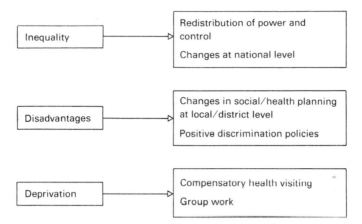

Fig. 3.5. Health visiting response to health needs.

viously. One approach is to use a matrix to plot client groups against social needs (Fig. 3.6).

The indicators used are those suggested in the following reports: Black Report (DHSS, 1980), Imber (1977), Belfast Areas of Special Needs (1976) and the Department of the Environment (1981). In this way there can be a targeting exercise to direct resources at those most in need.

We have to identify those needs which are amenable to action at

		Unemployed	Pensioners living alone	Social class V	One-parent families	Immigrant households
Social Need	Educational disadvantage					
	Personal handicap					
	Households lacking exclusive use of basic amenities					
	Private rented accommodation					
	Public sector housing					
	Overcrowded households					

Fig. 3.6. Matrix of need.

different levels. Clearly some needs can only be ameliorated at a national level, e.g. poverty, while others can be tackled at a local level – campaigning for a safe play area for children, for example. Action on health needs operates at four levels:

(1)   Macro or national level
(2)   District level
(3)   Professional level
(4)   Micro or community level.

   Workers have to be aware that there may not be a consensus on determining health needs. There may be no homogeneity of need, no agreed perspective, and little agreement on solutions.

Action on health needs

At a national level health visitors should be involved in attempting to influence policies affecting health. The following are some ways of doing this in conjunction with the local community:

(1)   Linking into national pressure groups, e.g. Child Poverty Action or Mencap.
(2)   Lobbying professional bodies such as Health Visitors' Association or Royal College of Nursing.
(3)   Sending letters to the national press.
(4)   Contacting Members of Parliament and Members of European Parliament; inviting them to discuss the issue, see local conditions, and meet the local people.
(5)   Preparing evidence to be considered by the District and Regional Health Authorities.

   At a district level, health visitors may be involved in the following ways by:

(1)   Establishing the evidence for discussion at the District Health Authority and contacting the Nurse member of the Authority.
(2)   Linking with other concerned professionals, e.g. social workers, community workers, district nurses and doctors.
(3)   Linking with voluntary groups and local pressure groups.
(4)   Contacting local newspapers and local radio.

Similarly, health visitors can also operate at a professional level by:

(1) Examining existing services to establish if they are responsive to need.
(2) Considering alternative strategies to delivery of health care, e.g. outreach schemes in shopping areas or providing a health worker whose main function will be to liaise with groups in the area.
(3) Discussing changes in role to meet health needs, e.g. developing an advocate role and acting as a linker/connector from the organization to the local community.
(4) Developing links with Community Health Councils.
(5) Asking for training in the activities which influence policy from organizations which provide refresher courses and in-service training.
(6) Maintaining an up-to-date community health profile.
(7) Providing the community with information about health care activities.
(8) Promoting self-help activities if appropriate.

In short, the health visitor can be an enabler, facilitator or catalyst for change by helping the local community to identify needs and provide strategies to ameliorate health problems. There are many examples of such health initiatives.

Having identified a community which, for example, has a low take up of services or multiple health problems, the health visitor could link with a range of other health, educational and social agencies to plan a 'health week' which could include:

(1) Local radio and newspapers running features on health issues.
(2) Schools undertaking health-related projects.
(3) Linking with voluntary groups such as Action on Smoking and Health to set up stalls in local shopping centre.
(4) Local factories having displays or features in the dining area and throughout the work place.
(5) Sports centres mounting a fitness competition.
(6) Youth clubs and youth groups having health discussions and projects.
(7) Street theatre presenting material with a health message.

In addition, the health visitor could:

(1)   Conduct a health phone-in.
(2)   Set up a health fair in the local clinic or community hall featuring,
      for example, stalls on nutrition and exercise – use could be made of
      videos on health issues such as smoking.
(3)   Set up health education stalls in local markets or shopping centres.
(4)   Set up health education displays in clinics, general practitioners'
      surgeries or any place where people wait – this could include bus
      stations, DSS offices and Job Centres.
(5)   Organize a series of workshops on health issues.

   Use your imagination. Do not be restricted by traditional methods of
service delivery. The emphasis should be on being where the clients are,
not making them fit into what is convenient for the professionals. The
issues that should be explored with the community include the following:

(1)   How do local people describe the need and what is the reality for
      them; do they, for example, describe the problems/needs in terms
      which show acceptance? Do they demonstrate that they have little
      belief in their ability to effect change or do they view the problem as
      amenable to action?
(2)   What is the extent of the problem/need, i.e. what is the size, scope
      and effect of the problem/need? It is important to be aware of any
      social values involved and of who stands to either gain or lose by
      effecting change. For example, if there is a problem concerning glue
      sniffing what is the implication of this for the local people and the
      shopkeepers?
(3)   What are the perceived origins of the problems/needs? It is very
      difficult to establish causation for many issues in community health
      but it is necessary to identify what the community sees as causative
      factors in order to focus the response, e.g. the need to provide a
      health education programme in schools to reduce road accidents.
(4)   Who in the community is interested enough to devote the time and
      skills to effecting change and act as a spokesperson for the
      residents? Do the spokespeople represent the community and are
      they representative of all the people? Do they share the values and
      consensus of the area?
(5)   What existing groups are there and how can they be utilized?

   One way of focusing on health needs is to use the principles of health
visiting as a framework (Fig. 3.7).

Principle	Example
Search for health needs	Identifying health-damaging behaviour such as inadequate diet or unrecognized depression
Stimulation of the awareness of health needs	Encouraging an individual to change health-damaging behaviour; encouraging local community to set up a group for isolated mothers
Influence on policies affecting health	Identifying a group with particular health needs and presenting a case to nursing management for a change in Service provision. This might be the establishment of a Well Women Clinic. Campaign for a change in housing provision.
Facilitation of health-enhancing activities	Providing the means by which clients can be helped, e.g. setting up a stress reduction clinic or a series of health talks for teenagers

Fig. 3.7. Principles of health visiting as a framework.

Models of participation

It is possible to present three models of participation which may be used in the community. These are:

(1) Marginal involvement
(2) Community-based initiatives
(3) Self-help activities

The marginal participation model

The marginal participation model still sees the professionals as experts and leaders. It recognizes that there is diversity within the community and accepts the involvement of community leaders as representatives of the community members. The important elements of this model are the need for effective communication between professionals and the community and the need to gain manpower and materials to improve health care resources. This can be achieved by using existing networks, establishing meetings, and involving the community in fund raising. The aim of such an involvement is to modify existing systems to meet local needs but the major influence still rests with the professionals.

Community-based initiatives model

The community-based initiatives model implies that lay people can influence health care delivery by shifting the power of decision-making. The role of the professional is to help people understand what they can do to improve health. It is more concerned with creating educational opportunities than creating structures and more committed to continuous involvement by the community. It focuses on process rather than content. This approach challenges the dominant role of the professional and suggests that they act as resources, not sources, of health care. The community can be motivated in two ways. Firstly, by teaching about health activities, the community can be motivated by realizing the problems and the possibilities of solving some of these problems. Secondly, by bringing the community into participation, they gain confidence and more self-esteem in defining their own problems and needs. This 'bottom-up' rather than 'top down' planning attempts to ensure health activities which service the community rather than the professional needs.

The danger implied in the above model is that problems will seem to be amenable to change by communities when in reality many problems need changes in the socio-political sphere of influence.

Self-help model

The self-help model is one that is often proposed as a 'trendy' solution to lack of resources. Like the word community, the term self-help is used as if it is always 'a good thing'. Yet in terms of health care the rationale of 'self-help' is a criticism of the professionals and their unwillingness or inability to help. Self-help promoters recognize the ability of people who share common problems to work together to raise money and materials, and to give emotional support and/or technical expertise. Many self-help groups use professionals for advice and assistance but the professional should be considered a group member first and a professional second.

Self-help groups define their own terms of reference rather than have them defined by experts. Self-help groups affect health care on a limited scale because they are essentially sectional in their approach and often represent only a small number of people in the community. They often act as pressure groups attempting to gain more resources for their cause. Self-help groups may also effect change by their very presence. The mere existence of public interest groups, and the knowledge that officials are being 'watched', affects behaviour quite apart from any particular action that such groups may take (Schuck, 1977).

Table 3.1 Models of community participation

Approach	Professional roles	Organizational changes	Motivation of participants
Marginal	Experts and leaders	Modification of existing systems	Influence on resource allocation
Community	Resource/facilitator	Restructuring of system	Shift in power base
Self-help	Peripheral	Structured from within group	Need for support for common problems

These three approaches have implications for professional roles and the organization (Table 3.1). It may be that visitors should develop these three models of participation. What is clear, however, is that we cannot be complacent about the existing level of participation.

Health visitor involvement in participation

Participation is a complex undertaking and we need much more analysis of what it would mean for the role of community health workers and the organization of the services. At present, there is little participation and emphasis paid to the concept. Even in the very obvious area of providing clinic services, how often do we ask clients what they would like? Should some pilot client/health visitor consultative schemes be set up in order to actively seek the views of those who use the services? A concerning example of how little we consult clients is when health visitors, as professionals of the primary health care team, conduct case conferences without asking families what they are capable of and want. To discuss the case of a demented elderly person, for example, in the absence of the relatives who will have the major responsibility of care is professional arrogance and, on behalf of our clients, should not be tolerated.

In terms of participation, the work of the health visitor has two main foci. One is to mobilize the residents concerning health issues: for example, in assisting in the formation of pressure groups. The second is to give people knowledge and skills related to health. Those most in need may be alienated from services and may only accept help from outside the statutory agencies. Health visitors should then be working through bodies such as the Workers' Educational Association or Community and Tenants' Groups. Working through local people may be one way of reaching those most in need, though professional hackles may rise at the suggestion of training lay women, for example, to help mothers with social and health problems.

If people are being helped in a way which is acceptable to them and will not accept statutory services, does it matter if the helpers are not highly trained professionals? Lay people, because of their knowledge from a community, know the context of health issues, can provide realistic alternative strategies for health care delivery, and can advise on priorities. Local people provide judgments about what is acceptable and give information on operational details. Health visitors, for example, work mainly with women (Dunnell & Dobbs, 1983) and in this sphere of work there is an increasing opportunity for participation.

Women and community – the case for participation

In many communities there is a discernible trend which is cutting across class and political groupings and that is the spontaneous *ad hoc* organization of women to meet a particular need or combine against a specific threat. This is evident in the range of self-help and protest groups which have been mushrooming in the last five to ten years. Examples of these are the Rape Crisis Centres, Women's Aid and Well Women Groups and Centres.

This development should come as no surprise to health visitors who must recognize that the matters women most care about, and are responsible for, are centred in the home, i.e. in the community (Bayley, 1982). This differs from the world of most men for whom the core of their life is work and the activities associated with that. Women are very aware that the community they inhabit is not the community idealized by politicians, but it is the place where women are in direct contact and confrontation with the State as represented by housing, welfare and health services. For many women, their contact with these services only reinforce their roles and make implicit and explicit the women's degree of failure.

Many of the early community development schemes ignored women's problems and a growing criticism of the treatment of women's issues has arise. Mayo (1977) sees that there was a tendency to reinforce sexist role stereotyping by concentrating on women as wives and mothers, and thus failing to facilitate the developments of other facets of their personalities or meet other needs and aspirations.

As an example of this, health visitors still lay insufficient emphasis on community involvement as it affects women. Many health visitors are involved in organizing mother–toddler groups but the functions of these groups is often little more than a reflection of middle-class values and views of women. Health visitors may therefore not be involved in consciousness raising or in encouraging action to ameliorate neglected issues such as the health problems of older women.

The fact that women themselves are organizing is indicative of their concern and their determination to bring about change. The women's health movement is a good example of how women have challenged the health care professionals and have spearheaded a nationwide movement. It is the case that in the North West of England, for example, there is a strong, articulate body of women who have succeeded in setting up women's health classes and self-help groups and have thus been instrumental in the establishment of Well Women Clinics. While these women are from very diverse backgrounds, they appear united in their demand for health care on their terms.

The Well Women Clinics which have been established in the Wythenshawe, Withington and Rusholme areas of Manchester are examples of how lay and professional women have changed policies and provided a very different clinic service from that of a cytology or family planning clinic. The emphasis is on helping women to identify their own health and social needs by taking a holistic approach. Women's health needs, after all, involve more than cervical smears and breast examinations. The women are invited to join a range of self-help groups and attend sessions on specific health problems such as depression.

The emphasis in the Well Women Clinics is on partnership between both the workers themselves and the clients. Every effort is made to involve the women who come in for their health assessment by demystifying health and medical practice. The three clinics in the Manchester area vary according to local needs and staff. They are, however, involved in training programmes for all workers and there is an emphasis on sharing skills and knowledge. The clinics are non hierarchi cal in organization with all decisions being made at monthly policy meetings. This means that all workers participate and have an involvement in evaluating and developing the clinic outside any rigid bureaucratic models. The professional workers do not have automatic authority because of their specialized knowledge. The clinics are therefore a reflection of what the local women want and this is made evident by the way the clinics are used and the high degree of satisfaction expressed by users.

The Well Women Clinics are an example of the move to partnership and reflect much of the current rhetoric about health care (Orr, 1988). These clinics are:

(1)   Concerned with prevention.
(2)   Meeting local and articulated needs.
(3)   Involving local communities and forming partnerships.
(4)   Using voluntary and lay helpers.
(5)   Based on a self-help ethos.
(6)   Reaching clients not covered by existing services.
(7)   Bringing together a range of disciplines.
(8)   Taking a holistic approach to care.

CONCLUSION

There is a growing dynamic and innovatory community health movement existing in the UK. The time is right for health visitors to contribute
to this movement and to develop practice. Without wishing to reflect on
some past golden age it is pertinent to draw parallels between the radical
community development work of our health visiting fore-sisters in the
latter half of the 19th century and the current community health
movement. The context is, of course, fundamentally different and the
beliefs may not be so diverse. As a group, health visitors have to decide
the emphasis of their work. It is recognized that there may be limitations
and latent dysfunctions which may accompany shifts in practice. We
operate in the realm of uncertainty but, given the current state of health
care, it is contended that health visitors should be used to facilitate the
development of their role in the assessment of community health needs
and to contribute to the development of the 'new public health'. Not all
health visitors will wish, or will need to work at a community level. There
has to be a degree of specialization within a team of health visitors. The
challenge for the future will be to match the different skills of health
visitors and other community health nurses with the identified needs of
individuals, families and communities.

4 Assessing Individual and Family Health Needs

Jean Orr

MODELS OF INTERVENTION IN FAMILY LIFE

The 'family' is the one institution in our society which is viewed as being important, not only for individual welfare but for the overall good of society. The family is used as a symbol in all discussions of social life and social welfare and it is seen as a necessary function of the state to intervene in family life through the provision of services and benefits. Health visitors are, more than most other health workers, involved in visiting families in their homes and in providing a unique service by working with families across all social classes, irrespective of any illness or crises. To work with families in this way gives health visitors considerable experience of family life and the tensions which are a normal part of living, thus placing health visitors in a privileged position to monitor social and economic policies affecting health. It is also a responsibility to work with individuals in this personal and important sphere of their lives.

The notion of intervening in family life to assess need is complex and has within it tensions based on the relationships between the State and the family. On the other hand, the family is seen as being a private and personal unit especially when there are no children and the dominant values of society are being upheld. The state, however, first intervenes in the family often when a woman becomes pregnant and always when the child is born. Reproduction is therefore seen as a legitimate point for intervention. Pregnancy and childbirth results in the private family becoming the public property of the professionals. After all, doctors often decide and legitimize when a woman is pregnant and decide on the availability of abortion if that is requested. The medical profession tends also to at least partly control contraception. Social workers on the other hand have a major role in deciding if children should be taken into care. The parents have to measure up to the professionals' expectations and current child rearing theories and the emphasis is mainly on reinforcing conformist types of family patterns. The focus is often on the woman's role in the family and it is women who find themselves on the interface

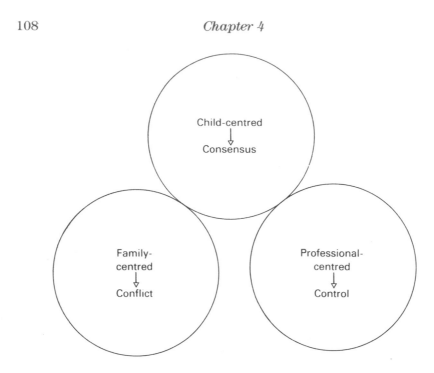

Fig. 4.1.   Models of intervention in family life.

with social and health services. The State is concerned about the role of women as mothers and care givers and emphasizes these roles to support the policy shift in community care. The State, however, is not so concerned about the social costs imposed on women within the family (Rimmer, 1983) and neither is it so concerned about women as women (Kiernan & Wicks, 1990). There is little emphasis on women's health outside the medicalization of child bearing and child rearing practices just as there is little concern with the health of men other than as workers or warriors.

✦ Three models of intervention in family life can be shown to exist (Fig. 4.1), the child-centred model, the family-centred model and the professional-centred model. ➤

(1)   *The child-centred model.*
      This model has strong historical credence and institutional support in other areas of social policy. The proper focus of services is seen to be the wellbeing of the young child, with other family members, especially fathers, playing secondary roles. This model is essentially one of consensus (Fig. 4.2).

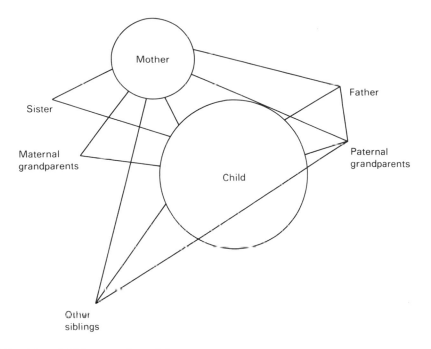

Fig. 4.2.   Child-centred model.

(2)   *The family-centred model.*
      While recognizing the importance of children, this mdoel tends to
      be more concerned with resolving conflicts within the family unit. It
      has the satisfactory functioning of the family as its main aim.

(3)   * *The professional-centred model.*
      There seems to be an emergence of a third model, the so-called
      professional-centred model. This means that as social and health
      policy changes towards community care there is more involvement
      and control, by professionals, in family life.

   The idea that families should care for their needy such as the
handicapped and elderly is not new (Rossiter & Wicks, 1982). The new
element is that the family unit and home is now seen as the desirable
place for care, not necessarily because it is best, but because it will soon
be the main, if not the only place. Professional community workers must
therefore use the home as a focus for their endeavour. This shift from
ward to bedroom or living-room raises questions about the role of
professionals in controlling family resources and actions in the name of

the State. With increasing specialization in health and social services there is a danger of fragmenting care. Each group of professionals tends to state their belief in the totality of the family unit and then proceed to segment and fractionalize it in pursuit of professional goals and status.

The family unit is being seen as the key learning environment for an increasing number of students of nursing, medicine and education. There is a growing interest in the family and community and a lack of debate about the ethics of using families to promote professional education. This model is based on a functionalist perspective and does not recognize any issues of conflict or dysfunction. There is little discussion of the issues surrounding the assessment of family need and little recognition of the value-laden nature of determining need.

THE CONCEPT OF NEED

The concept of need is absolutely fundamental to the understanding of social policy and the welfare state. The recognition and satisfaction of needs marks the social welfare function of the modern State from its other functions. Forder (1974) has argued that it is the concept of need that differentiates social welfare services from other types of institutions. While the concept may be of fundamental importance in social policy the issues and debates surrounding the definition and measurement of need are far from resolved. These are, however, fundamental to resource allocation in health care, as need is the most commonly used criteria for decision-making. This gives cause for concern when there is little available information on health needs (Lind & Wiseman, 1980). Without perhaps fully recognizing the ambiguity surrounding the concept of need, health visitors have identified two principles of health visiting, 'the search for health needs' and 'the stimulation of the awareness of health needs'.

The utilization of the concept of need is also found in the definition of health visiting stated in the Council for the Education and Training of Health Visitors' Principles Document (CETHV, 1977):

'The professional practice of health visiting consists of planned activities aimed at the promotion of health and prevention of ill-health. It thereby contributes substantially to individual and social well-being, by focusing attention at various times on either an individual, a social group or a community. It has three unique functions:

(1)   Identifying and fulfilling self-declared and recognised, as well as

      unacknowledged and unrecognised health needs of individuals
and social groups.

(2)   Providing a generalistic health agent service in an era of increasing specialisation in the health care available to individuals and communities.

(3)   Monitoring simultaneously the health needs and demands of individuals and communities; contributing to the fulfilment of these needs; and facilitating appropriate care and service by other professional health care groups.'

The word 'need', used in the above statements, makes explicit certain assumptions and beliefs and raises issues for the practice of health visiting – issues, it must be said, that are not faced by health visitors alone but which face all professional groups operating within the social welfare network.

The stated principles and definitions imply that:

(1)   Needs, both recognized and unrecognized, exist and should be met.

(2)   There are a multiplicity of needs.

(3)   There are necessary and consequent actions which will be beneficial.

(4)   Groups or communities have a homogeneity of needs.

(5)   Needs are measurable and the measurement is based on the principles of rationality.

(6)   There is a shared view of what is normal or desirable.

(7)   There can be a hierarchy of needs from which to order priorities.

(8)   Need and demand are interrelated concepts.

(9)   The health visitor should be active in searching for health needs and in stimulating an awareness of health needs.

When examining these nine points arising out of practice we oversimplify the essentially complex nature of the concept of need at this stage in our professional development. We talk of searching for health needs but we have not yet identified and fully discussed the issues involved. Further, we may have been rather naive in assuming that there is a shared sense of meaning among health visitors about what is meant by the concept of 'need'. Many other social welfare workers use the term in a similarly ill-defined way. The Seebohm Report (1968), for example, sees the personal social services as 'large scale experiments in ways of helping those in need'. The word need is not defined. In a legislative context needs are rarely defined with precision and although a local authority may have a duty to provide for those in need of care and attention, there may be no further guidelines given.

Epidemiologists have invested considerable efforts in endeavouring to define 'need' as a national basis for planning. This is a futile exercise as need is a useless concept fulfilling no function (Glass, 1976). While Acheson and Hall (1976) do not totally agree with Glass, they do say that need, while seeming to exist, eludes the clutches of those who attempt to define it. While it is easy to sympathize with this position, the basic difficulty underlying the definition of need is the value-orientated nature of such an exercise.

What is meant by need?

The concept of 'need' is employed to indicate a basic requirement for survival – we all need a minimum of food and warmth. It is also used to describe minimum standards which are necessary to obtain a certain quality of life such as housing. Need is social, relative and evaluative. It is social in being defined according to standards of communal life, relative in that its meaning will vary from age to age and from society to society, and evaluative in that it is based on value judgments. Need is a relative concept which is conditional on a multitude of factors such as culture, social and economic conditions, the availability of treatments, and the provision of services (Lind & Wiseman, 1980). Views about needs will continue to evolve and change over time, but we must specify the assumptions made about the measurements of needs, the value judgments which underpin them, and the role of health visitors in utilizing the concept of need.

The National Health Service has to meet and where possible modify certain needs experienced by the population. Decisions about which individuals or groups should be given priority are often about what needs should be met and how this should be done. In using the concept of need to determine priorities, professionals are acting as gate-keepers, limiting access to scarce resources. Most people have probably experienced this either from doctors, receptionists or from DSS offices. Professionals not only limit access, but also decide on allocation of certain resources. They decide whether a need exists in the first place and secondly the most appropriate manner in which that need can be met. This means that need can be used to refer both to an identified problem and to the help which is required to alleviate it. The former is referred to as diagnostic need and the latter as prescriptive need (Thayer, 1973). Obviously, in attempting to meet diagnostic need, some forms of help will be more appropriate than others. The same presenting problem may be associated with a variety of circumstances, each creating a different prescriptive need. Thus dietary insufficiency may create a need for direct financial assistance and/or a need for an educational programme for the individual depending on circumstances. When a need has been diagnosed, the provision of a particular form of help does not mean that the need has necessarily been met. Need can only be said to have been met when the help or service provided has brought about an intended change in the circumstances of the recipient.

Need as a criterion upon which to decide the ordering of priorities, is applied to two types of decisions:

(1)   Whether to allocate resources
(2)   What type of resources to allocate.

The decision will depend in part on the type of service available, e.g. if it is a universal service or one based on the notion of selectivity (Jones *et al.*, 1978).

Problems arise when clients are seen to be in need of other services and are referred by the health visitor. There may be insufficient resources in the other agency to meet the client's needs, and the health visitor has to seek alternative strategies. It may also be the case that the perceived need of the client varies between agencies. Health visitors, for example, are concerned with preventing family violence, but the social services department may not see this as a priority and may be slow in accepting the referral. Since a major function of health visitors is to refer clients to other agencies, these issues become the most problematic. In addition, with decreasing resources it is possible that health visitors may experience severe conflict between what they see as the client's need and the available services.

Adelstein (1976) presents the following five definitions of need and demand:

(1)   Health need, perceived

A health care need is perceived when an individual or family identify and acknowledge an abnormality which they know should be treated. They may take no action or may make use of informal agencies, e.g. see their local chemist, or contact the health service. Not all perceived need will be recognized by the health care workers.

(2)   Health need, unperceived

A condition that is unrecognized by the individual or the family but is potentially discoverable when a screening procedure is undertaken.

(3) Demand, stifled

Perceived health need that is not translated into overt demand due to bottlenecks in the provision of facilities.

(4) Demand, unmet

Requests for health care that have not been fulfilled. These are identified as waiting lists but will also include events where individuals' expectations have not been fulfilled.

(5) Demand, met

A health need, however identified, that has been handled by one of the branches of the health service.

In examining Adelstein's definitions, health visitors are faced with a problem in orientation. We are not toally concerned with abnormalities and this makes our definition of need particularly problematic. In addition, we are involved in initiating contact with many of our clients and have to face the issue of discovering needs which may not be met. If we assess the needs of a family or group, do we have a moral obligation to ensure that these needs are fulfilled? It is defensible to raise expectations which cannot be met? Thayer (1973) points out that where it is possible to assess diagnostic need it may not be possible by the same means to assess prescriptive needs. However, estimates of prescriptive need should always indicate diagnostic need. In other words, we should not point out a need for services without demonstrating the existence of circumstances which these services are intended to alter. Therefore, some approaches may be used to assess or estimate both diagnostic and prescriptive need while others will only be concerned with the former. For example, we may identify a family as being under stress because of insufficient income and be able to obtain increased benefits. Alternatively, if no additional money is available then we have only identified the problem without at the same time being able to offer help which would alleviate it. Such help could be given in money management and budgeting or in political action to increase benefits.

Bradshaw's taxonomy of need

A useful categorization of approaches to the measurement of social need has been developed by Bradshaw (1972). His is a four-fold classification of need based on the derivation of the criteria adopted for recognizing need, be it diagnostic or prescriptive.

Bradshaw's taxonomy of need employs four definitions:

(1) Normative needs
(2) Felt needs
(3) Expressed needs
(4) Comparative needs.

Normative needs

Normative needs are defined in accordance with some agreed standard. A desirable standard is laid down by the expert or professional and is compared with a standard which already exists. If an individual or group falls short of the desirable standard then they are identified as being in need. A normative definition of need is by no means absolute. It may not correspond with other definitions of need and, of course, different experts may have conflicting standards. It may be relatively easy to lay down standards for housing – where, for example, inside plumbing and electricity may be accepted as two standards of adequate housing – but it is more difficult to set standards in less tangible areas such as health without becoming involved in making value judgments. Thus normative definitions of need may be different according to the value judgments of differing experts. Furthermore, the idea of normative need demonstrates a particular view of service delivery in that it places the expert or professional at the centre of need assessment.

Difficulties are experienced in setting norms because of individual differences and differences in the use of resources. In the field of nutrition, for example, there are individual differences in absorption rates and in requirements for the maintenance of health. Perhaps even more important is the difficulty of setting the goal itself. To speak of a need is to imply a goal, a measurable deficiency from the goal, and the means of achieving the goal (Forder, 1974). But even in the field of nutrition, in which we could expect reasonable precision, this poses problems. We can easily identify diseases of deficiency or diseases of excess, but there is little knowledge about optimum levels of nutrition and often there is disagreement between experts on the outcome of research, e.g. the level of fat in the diet is the subject of current debate.

To illustrate some of these difficulties, in health visiting practice, for example, some authorities are determining schedules of visiting for young children and thereby setting a norm or standard. We can question how this standard was determined and who determined it. We can also ask if such a standard can be applied to other District Health Authorities. More importantly, we can ask if this standard meets the felt needs of clients (see below).

To examine need simply from the normative perspective undermines a whole contemporary movement in social policy. This movement places emphasis upon revealing felt needs through such means as participation programmes and community action. The rationale of such programmes is that those who feel the needs are in the best position to say what these needs are. The identification of need, therefore, becomes synonymous with want. When assessing need for service, people are asked whether they feel they need it. It seems reasonable to involve people and yet involvement is very limited; often professionals both assume that they know what is best for the client and consider that consultation is time consuming.

Felt needs

Felt need alone may be an incomplete measure because it is limited by the perceptions of the individual in that they may express a desire for a service without needing it, fail to recognize their own need, or assume that no solution exists which would be acceptable.

Expressed needs

Expressed need or demand is 'felt need' turned into action. Under this definition total need is defined as 'those people who demand a service'. There may be people, however, who do not turn felt need into demand or who are suffering from presymptomatic disease. Because of this, it is unsatisfactory to use waiting lists as a measure of unmet need. It is, however, valid to examine the existence of self-help groups, the demands for Well Women Clinics and the support for Community Health Councils as examples of expressed need.

Comparative needs

Comparative needs refer to the imputed needs of an individual or group not in receipt of services but similar in relevant characteristics to others receiving services. For example, if a person is in receipt of a service because of particular characteristics and another person also has these characteristics but is not receiving a service, then we can say that the second person is in need. This is an attempt to standardize provision, but provision may not correspond with need. In other words, if area 'A' is receiving more resources than area 'B', area 'A' may still be in need. This highlights the problem of defining significant characteristics for comparison. Often this definition of need is used as a crude rule of precedence to assess eligibility for selective social/welfare services. The use of this definition of need can represent a radical approach in that it is based on concepts of equality and equity.

Bradshaw presents a taxonomy of need in which he demonstrates the interrelation of the four definitions; need, for example, may be postulated by the professional and if we take the example of fluoridation of

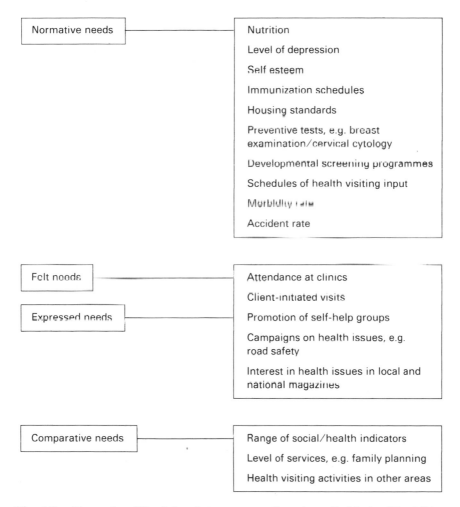

Fig. 4.3. Example of Bradshaw's taxonomy of need applied to health visiting.

water supplies, this was accepted by public health experts long before it was felt, demanded or supplied. The application of Bradshaw's taxonomy (Fig. 4.3) raises many issues for practice, not the least of which is the lack of clarity about what health visitors determine as normative need and what criteria we use in comparing provision in our areas with what is available in other parts of the district or country.

These concepts also raise questions about the allocation of resources across a wide range of families with which health visitors work. What is crucial to ideas of equality and equity is the prevailing belief that health visitors, as one example, should visit all social classes irrespective of the evidence that disadvantage is related to ill health.

Following the example of Bradshaw's taxonomy of need applied to seven studies of social welfare provision, Thayer (1973) concluded that this was a useful way to distinguish different approaches, despite the fact that criteria are closely interrelated and contain normative elements. In the case of felt need it may be a reflection of questions asked, or of the respondent's perception of what it is reasonable to expect. This will in turn be influenced by what is available. Expressed need obviously reflects what is available and the normative criteria controlling access to waiting lists. There will also be a normative element in the selection of relevant characteristics to use as comparative criteria. In other words the extent of measured need will vary. Normative need will vary according to the particular criterion adopted. Felt need will vary according to the observer's subjective assessment of intensity of feeling while the various channels through which demand can be expressed will give different estimates of expressed need. Comparative need will vary according to the areas which are considered and the particular social, demographic or environmental characteristics which are taken into account.

Value judgments

If the meeting of needs does specify the objectives of the health services then all that has to be done is for needs to be empirically discovered and then the health service can be made completely determinate and specified. If needs can be fixed in some straightforward, neutral, objective way then the goals of the health service could equally be fixed objectively, thus bypassing contestable appeals to social and political values. Questions about health services, and health visiting in particular, would no longer be questions about moral or political values but of matching means to needs and would therefore become a technical rather than an ideological problem. In addition, if this was possible it would enable us to measure the effectiveness of the health service by the criteria of met needs. However, according to Plant *et al.* (1980), the conception of need that is presupposed by this sort of view is that need is a non-normative concept. In other words, this supposes that needs can be discovered and articulated in an objective way by theorists, policy makers and health personnel. The evidence suggests this is not the case and the debate about needs' fulfilment remains central to social welfare provision and should be central to health visiting policy. Unfortunately, health visitors have been slow to treat the concept of need as problematic and many issues concerning needs are not debated within a health visiting context.

It is worth considering, for example, the question of the need for the provision of a community house for the mentally handicapped. It is necessary to assess whose needs are being met and by what criteria. It is possible to identify a number of interests. There are the policy makers who want to transfer resources, the voluntary bodies who support non-institutional care, the mentally handicapped themselves who may not even have been consulted, local residents who may be opposed to the idea, the community nursing and social work staff who may not have increased resources available, and so on. There are clearly conflicts of interest and need is based on the value judgments of the group involved. We may talk in a dispassionate way about the needs of groups or individuals, but in essence we are making value judgments and reflecting personal, professional and societal attitudes and preferences. The value-laden nature of needs' assessment is one we seldom consider and yet it is evidenced by the way we determine priorities. The very act of ranking need according to a hierarchy implies that there is a consensus regarding appropriate criteria of determining need. Due to the evaluative nature of the concept it is difficult to see how such consensus can exist. Yet the idea of ordering of needs to determine priorities implies that we operate just such a hierarchy in the teaching and management of health visiting. We do this as if it were a rational and value-free exercise.

If, for example, we talk about the health visitors' main priority - that of the young child - we are saying that this group is more worthy of attention than other groups in the caseload. On what basis do we make this judgment? It could be argued that as a professional group health visitors have not developed agreed and tested criteria for deciding such a priority.

In assessing community needs we are also faced with questions which concern values. Whose needs in the community have most salience? How do we balance the needs of, say, the unemployed with the needs of the elderly? How do we view the unemployed person who we know is working in the black economy? What is our position if we know that some of the families we visit are involved in crime? These issues are simply not debated even though they are part of the reality of community health work. Health visitors cannot work with such a wide range of the population and not be confronted with making value judgments about what are essentially moral dilemmas. Health visitors, for example, say that they are careful about what is recorded on infant cards because they recognize that information about family life may be detrimental to the child in school. If the clients are to have a greater role in participation in health care then health visitors will be faced with making explicit the value judgments which underpin how needs are determined. In particular, the words we use tell us a lot about how we view ourselves and our clients.

If, for example, we superficially examine the statement that we 'assess families and individuals' we see this as essentially being non-problematic and value-free. However, if we think about these words and substitute others with similar meaning we are faced with quite a different scenario. We can substitute the word 'assess', for example, with the following possibilities:

(1)   Judging families and individuals
(2)   Examining families and individuals
(3)   Measuring families and individuals
(4)   Weighing up families and individuals
(5)   Putting a value on families and individuals.

The assessment of families, therefore, can be seen to be a value-laden exercise.

If we replace the phrase 'families and individuals', we are forced to confront the following interesting alternatives:

(1)   Assessing our friends
(2)   Assessing our neighbours
(3)   Assessing our extended kinship network
(4)   Assessing our partners and colleagues
(5)   Assessing our fellow members of society
(6)   Assessing ourselves and nearest family.

What is conveyed by this exercise is the essentially judgmental and personal nature of working with families. It is impossible to avoid involvement in other people's lives and by implication, therefore, confronting issues in our own lives. We do not come to health visiting – or indeed any community health work - with a clean slate. All of us have experienced some form of family life, and this familiarity and expertise can be a strength and also a weakness. It is a strength in that we have some understanding of what goes on in families, how important they are, and how conflicts may exist which are never publicly expressed. The weakness is that our own experiences may be limited and biased. Any theoretical studies may serve only to reinforce our existing stereotypes and confirm our prejudices. Any tendency to see our own family experience as a standard from which to judge others constricts and colours how we see other families and how we make any assessment as health visitors operating within a professional perspective and involved in allocating resources.

Whose needs are being met?

There is often a difference between the professional and the client perspectives of what determines need. Most studies on social welfare provision concentrate on the professional role and there is little examination of the conflict which can be reality when resources do not meet need (Orr, 1983). For example, the clients' most pressing needs may be for decent housing or adequate benefits and in these spheres health visitors have little influence. It may be that to discuss health issues is desirable but the reality for many health visitors is that families must have their basic needs met before they can be concerned about changing existing habits which may be detrimental to their health.

Health visitors, for example, recognize the imperatives to help - with clothing, say, or household equipment - while at the same time recognizing that this may not be what they should be doing. These activities can be seen to be somehow less 'professional' than undertaking activities which have a veneer of professionalism such as developmental screening.

The dilemma for health visitors is that it is possible to identify so much need without demand. It has to be said, in the context of health visiting, that this is one of the strengths of the service in that health visitors' access to the general population enables them to articulate needs which may not be identified by any other group. Titmuss (1974) speaks of the existence of agents of social prevention within the social welfare services. He does not elaborate on this but it seems reasonable to assume that health visitors have little alternative but to identify social as well as health needs and to some extent be concerned with their amelioration.

Within this context, the concept of need is used in such a way as to make need different from wants, preferences and desires. It would be foolish to argue that social welfare services exist to satisfy people's wants and desires. The services exist to satisfy needs and this highlights the contrast which operates between wants and needs. It is often assumed that the economic market is where people seek the satisfaction of wants and preferences. Needs, and their satisfaction, characterize the social and health services although felt needs can be equated with wants. The situation with groups may be different. According to Plant *et al.* (1980), to ascribe a collective 'want' to a social group is to ascribe the same want to each member of that group. The case of needs statement is, however, said to be different in that to ascribe a need to a group does not necessarily involve the ascription of needs to each, or indeed to any, members of that group. Just as individuals come together in groups for many different reasons, individuals have different and conflicting needs which help them sustain difficult family relationships.

The family as a focus

It could be argued that working with families is what health visiting, as one example, is all about. While this is demonstrably true in terms of Government statistics, health visiting activity schedules and educational programmes, there are critical issues surrounding this aspect of health visiting which are little explored. The more we talk of being family visitors the more we expose our professional practice to criticism and scrutiny on this issue. Professionals cannot make repeated claims about themselves without recognizing that this places them in the vulnerable position of defending those claims. To simply say one is a family visitor raises fundamental questions which are not discussed by health visitors but instead are ignored and hidden within the taken-for-granted assumptions held by the professional.

In the first instance, one is struck by the implicit value judgment of the concept of being a family visitor and/or working with families. To work with families is seen somehow to be a 'good thing'. Like the word community, the word family is seldom used in a negative way. For example, we talk of being a family friend, restoring family values, maintaining the family unit and helping families to care for themselves. To complicate this further, the word family conjures up the image so beloved by advertisers of the working father, the stay-at-home wife, the two children and the dog. This is despite the reality of family life.

There have been many changes within the family unit and some of these are detailed below (Kiernan & Wicks, 1990):

- Only 8% of brides are teenagers.

- 26% of all children are born outside marriage (compared to 8% in 1971).

- 37% of recent marriages are likely to end in divorce.

- One in six families with dependent children are lone-parent families.

- One in eleven children under 16 have stepfathers.

- In 1901, 57 000 people were aged 85 or over - by the year 2001 the number will be over 1 million.

- 30% of women with children aged under 3 are in employment.

- In 81% of cases household washing and ironing is mainly done by the woman in dual-earner couples.

- 48% of women marrying for the first time has lived with their husbands prior to marriage - this figure was 7% in 1971.

- The average number of children per woman is 1.8.

- One in four young children will have parents who divorce.

- 98% of children live with their natural mothers.

- In 1901 one person in twenty was aged over 65; by 1981 it was one in seven.

- In 1975 60% of sixteen-year-olds left school and found jobs; by 1988 the proportion was 20%.

- 52% of married couples with dependent children are both in employment.

- In 1981 the number of centenarians stood at 2410.

Much of what is taught on health visitor courses fails to prepare practitioners to cope with the diverse patterns of the units in which people live. Deviations from the so-called 'normal' family unit are presented as problems needing special attention. Student health visitors appear to be encouraged to view the nuclear family as the norm and by implication therefore to measure all other groupings by this desirable standard. Can we be so sure that normal/nuclear families are problem free and that other types of family units are problem-centred?

Are we denying our own reality when we may have experienced other valid models of family constructs? Do the majority of health visitors themselves belong to the idea family unit? To what extent are they propounding an unrealistic model?

From whose perspective is the nuclear family being presented as an ideal? It may be that children who are the victims of incest or women who are the victims of violence within a family unit may not see the family as an essentially good institution.

There is a belief that any family is better than no family irrespective of the social costs. There is also the assumption that all members of a family benefit equally from membership and that the needs of each member can be reconciled with the overall benefits of the unit. Our life experience suggests that this is problematic but is little discussed in terms of how it relates to practice.

The needs of the woman, man and child within a family unit are not always consonant; neither are they always incompatible, nor static. The family shifts in structure and function over time and in relation to circumstance. Clearly, the needs of a new family with young children differs from the needs of a family with teenage children. The relationship between a woman and man is different before and after the birth of a first baby. There is difficulty in ascertaining whose needs are paramount within a family, to what extent family conflict is functional to the survival of the unit, and to what extent health visiting intervention will be welcomed and utilized.

The introduction of the Children Act (1989) certainly raises these issues; it is the most comprehensive piece of legislation yet framed about children and its purpose is to promote and safeguard the welfare of children. This must be the paramount consideration of the Court. The concept of parental responsibility replaces the phrase parental rights and sums up the duties, rights, powers and responsibilities and authority which a parent has in respect to a child and its property.

The belief underpinning this measure is the belief that children are generally best looked after within the family with both parents playing a full part and without resort to legal proceedings.

Defining needs, demands and wants

There are instances when individuals or groups do not identify themselves as being in need and yet can benefit from health care. Since they are unlikely to demand care unprompted their need must be articulated by a health care professional. An example of need without demand is a population which requires immunization against a potentially lethal infection. Another example is the need for prevention of respiratory tuberculosis, especially amongst immigrant groups. In essence, a considerable range of primary prevention is part of this need without demand. We identify, for example, children who are at risk from pre-natal and post-natal factors as being in need of surveillance. In this case there may be no demand. In fact, health visitors are largely concerned with identifying need without demand. Most other social welfare services operate on the basis of client initiation. Thus, we operate an outreach service which has explicit within it, the identification of unacknowledged needs and this is essentially the health visitor's professional function. It is also one of the main functions of the health visiting service and yet it is not without problems in terms of the client-professional relationship. After all, when someone seeks help from a doctor she has recognized a need for help or reassurance and should be relatively receptive to treatment or advice. This may not be the case in other situations when the client may not want to acknowledge needs and may reject the professional advice or health teaching. This is a difficulty in health promotion and in the uptake of preventive services.

The health visitor needs to understand what motivates individuals to change behaviour or to use preventive services. Rosenstock (1966) suggests that a decision to obtain a preventive or detection test in the absence of symptoms will not be made unless certain conditions are satisfied, as follows:

(1) The individual is psychologically ready to take action relative to a particular health condition. The extent of readiness to act is defined by whether the individual feels susceptible to the condition in question and the extent to which its possible occurrence is viewed as having serious consequences.
(2) The individual believes that the preventive test in question is both feasible and appropriate to use, would reduce either the perceived susceptibility to or the perceived severity of the health condition, and no serious psychological barriers to the proposed action are present.
(3) A cue or stimulus occurs to trigger the response.

Rosenstock then goes on to summarize three major principles.

(1) Preventive or therapeutic behaviour relative to a given health problem in the individual is determined by the extent to which the problems are seen as having both serious consequences and a high probability of occurrence, and the extent to which it is believed that some course of action will be effective in reducing that threat.
(2) Behaviour emerges out of frequent conflict among motives and among courses of action. Where motives themselves conflict or compete for attention, those that have the highest value of salience for the individual will actually be aroused.

(3)   Health-related motives may not always give rise to health-related behaviour and, conversely, health-related behaviour may not always be determined by health-related motives.

Finally, the health visitor has to understand the issues involved in utilizing the concept of need and how this links to working with families in a way that is understandable not only to the families but to the rest of the health services.

HEALTH VISITING PRACTICE

As community health workers, we make statements of our professional intent in such global terms as to be often meaningless. What do we mean by 'assessing family health' or assessing the physical, social and emotional health of families and individuals? We simply do not have the tools at present to undertake such an exercise. To state one's professional intent in such broad terms makes it impossible to produce meaningful criteria for health visitors to use. If we are not clear and concise about our professional intent we can be easily directed into activities which are peripheral. We can also reach out for alternative models of practice which hold promise of clarity, however spurious. Health visitors, for example, claim to have moved from a medical model but it is unclear what they have put in its place. It would seem that health visiting is almost being forced to absorb the nursing process as an answer to this vacuum and this has led to a growing concern and confusion over the transference of the nursing process to health visiting. The introduction of the so-called health visiting process as a management tool has led it to be seen as nothing more than a new form of record keeping which, it could be argued, reflects what has been happening in the record keeping of district nurses. Secondly, it has resulted in health visitors maintaining that the 'process' is what they have always done.

There is, as is often the case, a little truth in both of these statements but that does not make them totally correct. The view taken here is that the nursing process is a decision-making and problem-solving activity which is not unique to nursing but which can be found in many other areas as management, social work and education.

The use of a decision-making approach may very well mean a different style of record keeping and it should reflect what health visitors have been doing in terms of their work. A fundamental point is missing, however, and that is that any decision-making process does not happen in isolation. It should be firmly based within a theoretical framework

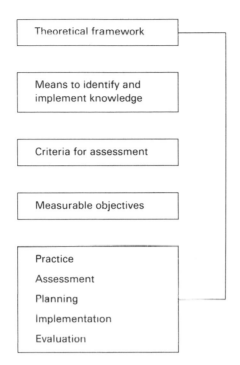

Fig. 4.4. Stages in determining health visiting practice.

from which we can determine the criteria for assessment and formulate measurable objectives (Fig. 4.4). In other words, we need a theoretical framework to determine the rationale of our work and what our assessment criteria should be. If health visitors wish to call what they do the health visiting process then that is their choice. Here this decision-making process will be identified as health visiting practice and the concentration will be on exploring issues of theory rather than the semantics.

Theoretical aspects

Riehl and Roy (1980) define a theory as 'a scientifically acceptable general principle which governs practice or is proposed to explain observed facts'. A theory is said to be at a deeper level of reality representation than a model. A model may represent structure while theory denotes function. In health visiting, as in the rest of nursing, we are beginning to recognize the need for developing theories and models which provide the basis for selecting knowledge to be used in education and which will provide a framework for practice. A theory may be derived either deductively or inductively. That is to say we can follow the deductive method and select relevant concepts from other bodies of knowledge such as sociology to examine and explain situations, or, alternatively, we can follow the inductive approach which starts with the experience and proceeds to develop concepts from the health visitor's reality. In this chapter our interest in theories and models is to provide a prescription for action (Riehl & Roy, 1980) and therefore all theory should be chosen with its practice implication as the most essential criterion.

The following four levels of theories in a practice discipline are put forward by Dickoff *et al.* (1968):

(1) *Factor isolating theories* – these involve naming and classifying.
(2) *Factor relating theories* – these involve depicting or describing and relating factors, and therefore give a natural history of the subject, e.g. anatomy.
(3) *Situation relating theories* – concerned with causal relationships and therefore allow for prediction which is essential for problem solving.
(4) *Situation producing theories* – these are prescriptive theories and are the most mature level of all theories and are comprised of:
   ● specifying the goal to be achieved
   ● surveying alternatives
   ● choosing among alternatives
   ● prescribing activities to attain the goal

Dickoff *et al.* suggests that the elements to be examined in determining any model of nursing are:

(1) *Agency:* who or what performs the activity?
(2) *Patiency or recipiency:* who or what is the recipient of the activity?
(3) *Framework:* in what context is the activity performed?
(4) *Terminus:* what is the end point of activity?
(5) *Procedure or process:* what is the guiding procedure, technique or protocol of the activity?
(6) *Dynamics:* what is the energy source of the activity, e.g. physical, chemical or psychological?

This list may appear to be rather abstract but if we apply it to a health visitor working with an elderly person we may see its usefulness.

(1) *Agency:* health visitor
(2) *Recipiency:* elderly person
(3) *Framework:* functional assessment
(4) *Terminus:* determine health/social need and identify risk factors
(5) *Procedure:* questioning, listening, examining, screening
(6) *Dynamics:* physical, social, mechanical

The above elements form the outline of health visiting activity irrespective of the theoretical underpinning, and this helps us to concentrate on
the practice of health visiting in concrete and operational terms. At this
stage, we should consider the theoretical underpinnings which inform
our practice.

Such a scheme does not imply a consideration of theory in an abstract
or obtuse manner but enables questions to be raised about the basic
assumptions of what health visitors do. As health visitors, we take part in
a 'health visit' but what do we hope to achieve and what are the unique
elements of this health visit? Are we concerned with helping clients
towards self-care, are we attempting to help families cope with stress
and adapt to life changes? Do we see ourselves helping families to
manage their life crises and circumstances or are we concerned with
monitoring developmental stages?

These questions at one level seem very obvious but it could be argued
that without some clear statements of intent, health visitors appear
confused about their discrete function. It is conceptually inappropriate
to embrace only one theory. Just as in other social science disciplines
students are exposed to a range of theoretical positions, so must health
visitor students manage a range of different perspectives which will
provide different professional intents.

Health visiting draws on many disciplines to inform practice, and in
this respect it is similar to nursing. It is therefore useful to examine
relevant theories from nursing which could illuminate function. The
general orientations of these theories are transferable but may not
achieve a perfect fit, and we need much more work in this area. However,
as a preliminary step, it is useful to examine six nursing theories and
ascertain how they view the individual and what their goals and activities
are (Table 4.1). Further details of these theories are given by Riehl and
Roy (1980), Roy (1976) and Orem (1971).

Self-care and stress theories

Nursing theories can be classified into the following three types (Reilly,
1975):

Table 4.1   Outline of six nursing theories

Johnson (Behavioural systems model)	Rogers (Unitarian model)	Roy (Adaptation model)
View of the individual		
A behavioural system of 8 sub systems: 1 affiliative 2 achievement 3 dependency 4 aggressive 5 eliminative 6 ingestive 7 restorative 8 sexual	A unified whole possessing integrity and manifesting: 1 wholeness 2 openness 3 a capacity for abstraction and using language, thought, sensation and emotion	A bio-psycho-social being in constant interaction with a changing environment and having 4 modes of adaptation: 1 physiological needs 2 self-concept 3 role function 4 inter-dependence
Goals		
To bring about the individual's behavioural stability	To promote harmony between the individual and the environment with the ultimate goal of reaching the highest state of health possible	To promote adaptation in the 4 adaptive models
Activities		
To assess behavioural stability, decide on the dynamics of behavioural instability, intervene by restricting, defending, inhibiting or facilitating behaviour and evaluate that resulting behaviour	To gather data about the individual in the environmental field and to use technical activities, manual skills or human relations to repattern the individual and environment	To assess client behaviour and factors which influence adaptation levels and to intervene by manipulating the influencing factors (focal, contextual and residual stimuli)

Orem (Self-care model)	Newman (Stress model)	Chrisman (Developmental model)
The individual has a need for self-care action on a continuous basis to sustain life and health, recover from disease or injury and cope with their effects	The individual in a state of wellness or illness is a dynamic composite of the interrelationship of 4 variables: 1 physiologic 2 psychologic 3 socio-cultural 4 developmental The variables are always present and subject to stressors	The individual exists within a framework of change: birth, growth and development, maturation and death are integral parts of living. The individual can be viewed at any point in time as a unit of interlocking biological, interpersonal and intrapersonal and intrapersonal systems which are open to the environment and subject to change
To promote self-care activities	To provide a unifying focus for examining the individual, group or community's relationship to stress	To aid the individual's development along the life continuum.
Giving human assistance adapted to specific human needs and limitations in order that self-care activity can be maintained to sustain health and prevent ill-health	To provide nursing intervention at primary, secondary or tertiary levels to aid an individual's, group's or community's adjustment to stress which could affect optimal functioning	To analyse the client's biologic, interpersonal and intrapersonal systems. To analyse the interactions of these systems and relationships among the systems, time and the environment in order to support and promote health.

(1)   Systems theories such as the Newman's stress or Roy's adaptation
(2)   Developmental theories such as Chrisman's
(3)   Life process theories such as Rogers'.

For health visiting, the most appropriate theories are Newman's stress theory and Orem's self-care theory. Self-care according to Orem is the practice of activities that individuals personally initiate and perform on their own behalf in maintaining health and wellbeing. If we develop the self-care concept it will result in educating the individual to maintain or improve the state of wellbeing. Certain factors have been isolated as affecting the provision of self-care; age and health, for example, generally determine the amount of self-care activities a person can perform. An individual's established pattern of responding to external and internal stimuli will affect the decisions and actions relating to self-care. Values and goals are also likely to affect the selection of and performance of self-care action in health or in ill-health. Therefore self-care measures which are compatible with the goals and values held by the person will be dependent upon individual judgment and ability to perform them. Milio (1976) sums up the problem by stating that 'if it is agreed that health promoting life patterns are a good thing then focus for changing behaviour should be on the problem of how to make health damaging choices more difficult.'
Self-care action can be regarded as both positive and practical, involving decision-making and choice even with such activities as personal hygiene and food selection unless these have become habitual. Some health care techniques may be learned by specialized education or may be developed through practical experience in using certain techniques. Some individuals may choose to adapt themselves to the constraints imposed by chronic illness than develop and learn therapeutic measures of self-caring. Self-care is concerned with practices which are therapeutic and should achieve the following:

(1)   Support in life processes and promoting normal functioning
(2)   Maintenance of normal growth development and maturation
(3)   Prevention, control or cure of disease processes and injuries
(4)   Prevention of or compensation for disabilities.

Self-care can be seen to be necessary by all individuals at all times and Orem calls this 'universal health care'. In addition, self-care may be necessary in the event of injury, disease or exposure to infection. This is called 'health deviation care'. Health deviation care promotes the questions 'what is wrong?', 'why is this happening?' and 'what should I do?' Knowledge is essential in the management of health deviation. Self-care knowledge will be about what to do in a particular situation and how to carry out self-care activities.

Four groups for self-care are suggested, concerned with the following:

(1) *Rehabilitation.* Self-help is primarily concerned with helping individuals to adjust to their new situations through interaction with others who have undergone similar experiences, in order to develop coping techniques.
(2) *Behaviour modification.* Examples of this include groups such as Alcoholics Anonymous, weight-watcher groups, and anti-smoking groups.
(3) *Primary care groups.* This is not seen as a curative area but is concerned with chronic care assistance in adjusting to a lifestyle imposed through having a chronic condition.
(4) *Prevention and case findings.* Self-help organizing techniques are used in detecting alterations in health and wellness, e.g. breast awareness and monitoring programmes for hypertensives.

The Newman stress model is of particular interest to health visitors because its aim is to assist individuals, families and groups to attain and maintain a maximum level of wellness by purposeful interventions. These are aimed at a reduction of stress factors which are detrimental to optimum functioning. The concept of stress and the means of helping people deal with stress can be seen as the raison d'être of working with families.

What is meant by stress and how can the practitioner apply the concept. The concept of stress is primarily derived from physiology but it is now being used in a wider sense to mean disruption in personal, social and cultural processes that bear some relationship to health and disease. Friedman (1981) examines the concept of stress and points out that stress is always present in individuals and is intensified when there is a change or threat with which the individual must cope. This highlights three factors:

(1) Stress is always present
(2) Change as well as threat intensifies the stress
(3) The individual has to attempt to deal with the stress, in other words 'to cope'.

The factors or agents which cause an intensification of stress are called 'stressors'. Individuals can be stressed by such stressors as pain, infection, anxiety or unpleasant treatments, but stress can be caused by pleasant events such as having a baby or going on holiday. Individuals suffering from stress exhibit what has been called the 'general stress syndrome'.

General stress syndrome

The 'general stress syndrome' has three stages:

(1)   Alarm stage

This is an instantaneous, short-term, life preserving and wholly sympathetic nervous system response when the person consciously or unconsciously perceives a stressor and feels helpless, insecure or biologically uncomfortable. This stage is typified by a 'fight or flight' reaction. The person is ready to act, is more alert and able to adapt.

(2)   Adaptation or resistance stage

This is the body's way of adapting to the disequilibrium caused by the stressors, e.g. the body's temperature adjusts to excess heat. Exposure to minor repeated stress may facilitate adaptation but diseases of adaptation may occur, e.g. hypertension.

(3)   Exhaustion stage

This stage occurs when the person is unable to continue to adapt. This could be because the stress is prolonged, repeated too quickly or the person has poor coping mechanisms.

The health visitor is concerned with promoting the above 'resistance stage' and preventing or reversing the 'exhaustion stage' by crisis intervention, medical treatment, information giving or social action. Ideally the health visitor should be able able to identify potential stressors that the client may encounter and determine how to alter the stressors and best support the client's adaptive mechanisms.

There is an increasing awareness that stress is caused by an event which brings about changes in the life of an individual and is not always detrimental to the individual. We all need some degree of stress to motivate us to perform a task we may dislike. Some complex tasks such as formulating new theories of nursing may best be done when one is at a low level of arousal. We may, therefore, be suffering from stress but are we at the same time anxious?

Although the terms stress and anxiety are used interchangeably they are not the same. Anxiety is the psychological response to excessive unchannelled energy resulting from the stress reaction; it is a vague diffuse feeling of dread, uneasiness or general discomfort resulting from perception of a threat to the self, real or imagined.

Health visitors need to be aware of what coping mechanisms individuals have to deal with stress. If the crisis or stressful event is managed by effective coping the individual learns new coping behaviour and strengthens the emotional and problem-solving ability. If insufficient or inadequate coping methods are used deterioration in psychological functioning is likely. Coping tends to be related to the individual's appraisal of both the stressful event and the coping method. Coping behaviours can be long-term or short-term. Short-term methods include drinking alcohol, sleeping, eating, taking drugs or crying. Long-term methods include seeking help from friends or professionals, making plans to handle the situation or taking some definite action to alleviate the situation.

The short-term measures tend to be detrimental to long-term mental health, the long-term measures include realistic and constructive ways of coping with stress and dealing with the reality of the situation. How might stress be identified? The following are early signs of stress:

(1) Altered sleep pattern
(2) Inability to concentrate
(3) Tiredness
(4) Physiological changes, e.g. skin change
(5) Self-concept may change, e.g. the client may experience sexual difficulties
(6) Role failure may occur, e.g. the client may exhibit dependent behaviour
(7) Personality may alter, e.g. the client may become angry, guilty or depressed.

The health visitor should attempt to assess the client to ascertain whether the following is the case:

(1) Stress is real or imagined, e.g. does the client feel stressed because of lack of information about a condition?
(2) Response is adaptive or maladaptive, e.g. crying may be a very

adaptive response in a grief situation but not if it was to occur over a long period of time

(3) Response is mild, moderate or severe, e.g. are the physiological changes inhibiting normal functioning?

The health visitor will assess whether the stressors are seen as noxious or not depending on the following:

(1) Intra-personal factors, e.g. responses inside the body
(2) Inter-personal factors, e.g. role expectation
(3) Extra-personal factors, e.g. social and cultural considerations.

In a stress situation the health visitor should help the client to recognize stress and to gain insight into causes and should help the client cope with the stress in constructive ways, e.g. long-term coping behaviour depending on whether the stress can be dealt with, removed or reappraised.

The health visitor is involved in the recognition of stressors or potential stressors, the strengths and weaknesses of the client, and in the recognition of the reaction to and recovery from stress. The intervention may be as follows:

(1) *Primary:* to reduce possible encounter with stressors, e.g. give information to reduce anxiety
(2) *Secondary:* to relieve stress which is present, e.g. helping client to obtain social security benefit
(3) *Tertiary:* this could follow when equilibrium has occurred and, for example, could take the form of education to prevent recurrence of a problem.

The above is a brief outline of one way that a nursing model can be used.

The following assessment schedule has been drawn up based on the concepts of self-care and stress. Health visiting could usefully develop a theoretical perspective which has a framework of the Newman stress model with the main goal being self-care.

Health status assessments

The health status assessment (Fig. 4.5) has at its epicentre clients' perception of their health needs, problems and resources. Its objectives include:

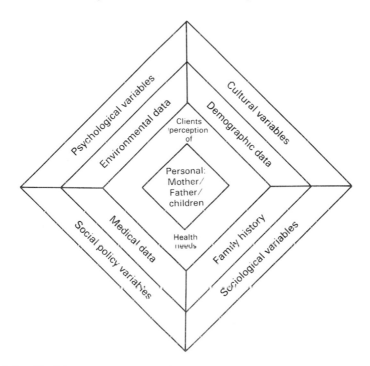

Fig. 4.5.   Health status assessment.

(1)   Determining the extent to which the individual has achieved optimum wellness.
(2)   Ascertaining the level of functioning in relation to their own lives and within the family group.
(3)   Identifying the existence of past and present stressors and coping mechanisms.
(4)   Ascertaining the existence of self-care skills of individuals and their social networks.
(5)   Identifying health-damaging behaviours, environmental and genetic factors.

From the way in which assessments schedules are written there is an assumption that the health visitor moves smoothly through the questions and that there is a logical progression through the topics to be discussed (Table 4.2). The reality is very different and there has to be a recognition that any assessment schedule is a tool or a means to enable the clients to talk about themselves, ask questions, and let them consider and discuss areas of their health that they may not have considered. The

Table 4.2   Health status assessment schedule

Demographic data

- Name
- Age
- Sex
- Marital status
- Race/religion

Family history

- Family structure
- State of health of family
- Client's role in family, e.g. mother, granny
- Interaction patterns and problems with social networks
- Member of family with most influence in health care matters
- Links with community

Medical history

- Pathological variables: present/past illness; present medical regime; future medical plans
- Biological variable: restrictions of functioning due to maturation or genetic defects
- Immunization status

Environmental data

- Living situation: housing; social climate
- Hazards to health and development
- Availability of recreation
- Availability of health care facilities

Cultural/sociological variables

- Socio-economic groups
- Economic status
- Role (distance, conflict, mastery, ambiguity)
- Function
- Education level
- Values/beliefs: in particular with regard to health, child care and use of health services such as family planning
- Present versus future orientation
- Communication patterns

Psychological variables

- Cognitive state and level of perception
- Level of stress and coping mechanisms
- Self-concept
- Self-esteem
- Interdependence: dependence; loneliness

Table 4.2   Continued

Social policy variables

- Contact with other agencies
- Use of health care facilities, e.g. baby clinic
- Use of social service provision, e.g. day centre
- Nature of social welfare benefits
- Nature of expressed or unexpressed need

Client's perceptions of:

- Major problems/needs
- How the client may cope with their problems/needs
- What self-help measures may be taken
- What help is available from the family, friends or care givers

---

assessment is not an end in itself but rather it is a means to an end. In addition, there is a danger that the concentration on seemingly objective assessment schedules will result in a spurious and pseudo objective outcome. It is possible to think that the more facts we have the more we will be able to identify with our clients. Of course, there are certain indicators which help us to understand the families but there has to be a recognition that facts will not help us to deal with the emotional 'here and now of clients'. It may be that health visitors rely on facts to prevent them getting involved in feelings and emotional situations. It is not always the case that if we know more about clients in terms of social or health indicators we know more about them as unique individuals.

HEALTH VISITING PRACTICE

This has four main components:

(1)   Assessment of health status
(2)   Planning of health visiting
(3)   Implementation of health visiting
(4)   Evaluation of health visiting

Assessment of health status

Health status assessment involves the following three stages:

(1)   The health visitor will collect data about the individual or group in

order to determine individual or group needs, problems and
resources. The emphasis is not solely problem-centred but must
involve looking at actual and potential need. In addition, it is also
necessary to identify resources which are available to the individual
and group, be those resources located in social networks, the local
community, or from within the person themselves.
(2)   The next stage is to enable the client to articulate his/her own
       needs, and to establish whether these needs are recognized by the
       rest of the social network.
(3)   The final stage is to analyse, interpret, compare and synthesize this
       range of information in order to compile an assessment which
       adequately represents the needs, problems and resources of the
       individual.

   There may be a range of outcomes from this assessment; ten examples
of needs' analysis are described here:

(1)   No need exists, the individual's state of wellness is affirmed and
       periodic reassessment will be planned at specific intervals linked,
       for example, to developmental stages or to life change events.
(2)   No need exists but a potential need may be offset, e.g. by giving
       information. This is the primary stage.
(3)   A need exists but this is being handled successfully by the
       individual, or other agencies, and periodic reassessment will be
       planned.
(4)   A need exists for which the individual requires help in coping. This
       help may be the giving of information, providing support or
       counselling, obtaining resources, or referral to other agencies.
(5)   A need exists which the client cannot cope with and intervention
       is required for a short time, e.g. dental caries. This is the secondary
       stage of prevention.
(6)   A need exists which must be monitored over a long period of time,
       e.g. child abuse.
(7)   A need is imposed unexpectedly upon the individual and crisis
       intervention is required, e.g. sudden homelessness or severe home
       accident.
(8)   A need exists which is long-term and permanent and for which the
       individual requires some help. An example of such tertiary
       prevention is the existence of a chronic handicapping condition.
(9)   There may be outcome in which the perceived need of the
       individual and those of the professional are in conflict. For
       example, there may be evidence of child abuse which is denied by

the parents. In addition, there may be an identification of need by either the health visitor or the individual which is seen as not valid by the other. For example, an overweight toddler may cause concern in the professional but may be thought acceptable by the mother.

(10) There may be conflicts between the needs of individuals within the family unit, e.g. an isolated mother may demand more time from her husband than he is prepared to give.

Planning

Based on the completed assessment the health visitor will select from a range of alternative strategies and order these into a plan. This phase involves joint goal setting, ordering priorities and designing methods to meet the needs, alleviate the problems and utilize the resources of the individual, the group and the community.

Planning together with the individual involves the following:

(1) Assigning priorities to the needs of the individual
(2) Differentiating needs which could be resolved by:
   ● Individual or social networks
   ● The health visitor
   ● Other agencies.
(3) Designating specific actions to immediate medium-term and long-term goals and desired outcomes
(4) Recording needs, actions and expected outcomes.

Implementation

This phase is the operationalization of the plan. It involves the initiating and completing of strategies which will lead to the achievement of defined goals. This will be reassessed as the plan is activated.

Evaluation

This important phase involves the measuring of outcomes of the plan against the stated goals and will be discussed in Chapter 5.

An important feature of assessment is to identify to what extent individual needs are recognized and validated by others and what means are available to meet these needs. We can see how this might be examined in an individual need analysis (Table 4.3), which takes the example of a mother whose child has had a home accident.

Table 4.3 Individual need analysis

Individual	Perceived need	Recognized and validated by others in network	Means by which needs are to be met
Mrs Jones	Loss of self-confidence in mothering ability following child's home accident.	Husband — no Mother — yes Sister — yes	1 Discussion with husband 2 Advising relatives to reinforce mothering competency 3 Reinforcement and reflection of feeling from health visitor and other contact agencies

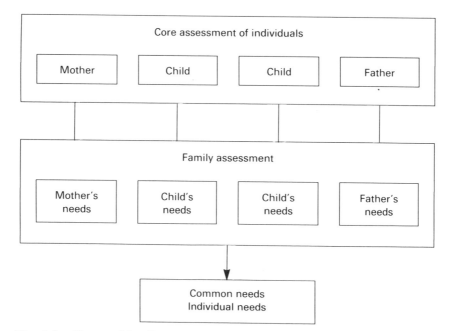

Fig. 4.6. Core and family assessment.

Core assessments

The recognition that individuals within the family group may have different and conflicting needs means that what may be required is a core assessment for each individual. These could then feed into a total family assessment without losing sight of individual positions (Fig. 4.6).

As an example of what is meant by core assessment it may be useful to apply this concept to the health needs of women. The work of Spencer *et al.* (1982) on the health needs of women suggests that an assessment should be carried out on a yearly basis and it is further argued here that this assessment should include physical examination, e.g. pelvic examination. The evidence also supports the view that health education is most effective when carried out in conjunction with a full health assessment. Health visitors should be encouraged to devise their own approach to this type of assessment but the following areas are suggested in the light of the needs demonstrated at Well Women Clinics (Table 4.4).

The entries for general physical health, lifestyle, social activities and relationships can also be used for men. There is little emphasis on men's health and, unlike women, they have not demonstrated particular needs, although the mortality and morbidity evidence suggests that men have

Table 4.4 Core health assessment

General physical health	Lifestyle	Social activities and relationships	Women's wellness
Current state	Level of nutrition	Support systems	Menstruation
Current treatment	Weight	Sense of isolation	Pre-menstrual
Illness/accidents In last year	Smoking	Control over life	tension
	Drugs	Enjoyment of life	Menopause
Concerns with	Alcohol	Stressors and	Vaginal health
1 digestive system		coping	Cystitis
2 bowels	Exercise	mechanisms	
3 skin	Rest/recreation		Breast
4 reproduction		Depression	examination
5 urinary	Stress reduction		
6 dental	Work hazards		
7 headaches			
8 sleep	Contraception		
9 others	Sexual functioning		
Preventive screening	Reproduction		

particular needs such as the prevention of cardiovascular disease. The reproductive function of women is highlighted but little attention is paid, for example, to male problems of impotency or scrotal cancer. Thus, what is suggested is that core health assessments are undertaken at regular intervals. Focusing health visitor intervention in this way would involve clients more actively in addressing their health needs and would enable the health visitor to achieve a more structured approach to her work.

FOCUSED INTERVENTION: THE CHILD DEVELOPMENT PROGRAMME

An example of focused work with families is being undertaken by the national Child Development Programme, based at Bristol University (Barker, 1984; Barker & Anderson, 1988). This programme was supported by the Bernard Van Leer Foundation of The Hague. It is a large scale intervention study which involves health visitors and it focuses on altering the human environment surrounding the disadvantaged child during the earliest years of life.

There are five basic elements in the study:

(1)   It concentrates entirely on influencing the immediate environment of the child rather than working directly with the child.
(2)   Both the principal and secondary caretakers in the child's environment, the mothers and fathers, have been encouraged to seek their own solutions to the problems of child rearing with help and advice, rather than direction, from the health visitors.
(3)   The concepts and strategies used are simple, down to earth, and relevant to parents.
(4)   Large scale and rigorous monitoring has been undertaken to assess the quality of the reported achievement.
(5)   Changes hae been made to the structures and functioning of the health visitors involved.

The study started in 1981 by obtaining the collaboration of six urban health authorities in England, Ireland and Wales; a total of 1031 families were involved with a total of 1051 infant children. These families were recruited by health visitors and were randomly selected from disadvantaged areas within the six authorities. The parents of 678 children received monthly intervention visits from their health visitors for periods of up to two years. The parents of the remaining 373 children served as controls for a comparison of the effects of the intervention. Five project interviewers carried out comprehensive assessment of the home environment and children's development so that all parents and children, both intervention and control, were assessed three times at yearly intervals. The intervention health visitors were given an initial nine-day training course and were seen individually and in groups for discussion of cases and for further in-service training in the developed principles underlying the project.

The initial visit

There are no set programmes or formal lists of behavioural goals for either the parents or the children. The health visitors have been trained to approach parents flexibly, discussing with them methods of stimulating the development of the children and how to overcome any development problems. The visit focuses on seven fields of development, namely:

(1) Language
(2) Social development
(3) Cognitive development
(4) Pre-school educational development
(5) Nutrition
(6) Health
(7) General development

Each health visitor is given a large range of cartoon material with accompanying guides covering the particular areas involved (Appendix 6). Three of these cartoons are used as one of the focal points of the visit. The parents can study them in depth between visits. The health visitor completes a record of social and health conditions and also records the extent to which the mother has carried out the developmental tasks agreed at the previous visit. A new set of development tasks is discussed during the visit, with the mother/father being encouraged to put forward her/his own ideas for the coming months. The agreed tasks are recorded and given to the mother to remind her of what has been planned.

Health visitors are encouraged to focus on areas needing extra stimulation: for example, if there is too little language development, activities might be suggested in which the mother regularly placed herself and the child in a natural situation - at a window, for example - where intensive one to one communication can occur between mother and child as they watch the traffic and people pass by. The emphasis is on seeking solutions to problems which are both acceptable to the mother in her environment and developmentally useful.

The second phase

Following evaluation of the first phase of the project it was felt that because of the many demands placed on health visitors by other work pressures such as clinics and crisis intervention, some health visitors should be allocated to enable them to concentrate full-time on the support, education and guidance of primiparous parents. In other words, one out of every three to five health visitors should become first-parent visitors, with their colleagues undertaking other family visiting and carrying out structured intervention visits to those multiparous families facing particular difficulties. They should also take on a wider public health role.

The first-parent health visitor visits ante-natally and post-natally at monthly intervals (or more frequently if necessary in the early months). She hands over the family to the generalist health visitor colleagues at about eight months. Up to half the families are kept on for a further period (a minority for up to three years), if it is judged that they need continued support. Where possible, families which are handed over receive three-monthly support visits from the general health visitors. Essentially, the first-parent visitor specializes in working with new parents to the exclusion of all other health visiting duties. The main programme content is the support and guidance of all first-time parents in the participating areas, and the subsidiary programme offers support and guidance to a selection of those parents (in the same area) who are bringing up two or more children in the face of serious social or other problems.

The concept of a first-parent visitor will raise fundamental questions about the role of the health visitor and will lead to an ongoing professional debate, particularly now that the project's second phase is in the process of being evaluated.

Many health visitors may say that the aim of this study is similar to what they are already doing. Although the programme stresses that this type of intervention is the nub of health visiting, there are quite crucial differences and emphasis in the study which all health visitors may benefit from examining. While little is formally prescribed, there is a structured framework within which the health visitor can work and adapt to individual circumstances. The health visitor is provided with considerable substantive material, e.g. a home visiting manual on the concepts of parent support which contains background material in each area of the programme. There is also a manual of cartoon sequences covering a variety of typical situations faced by parents from which the health visitor can select and order sheets of cartoons. This material is intended to promote discussion between the parents and health visitor.

For the ante-natal mother and parents of new born babies there are cartoons dealing with the health and nutrition of the baby and mother followed by cartoons dealing with early language development, social and other forms of early development. For the parents of infants, toddlers and pre-school children there are cartoons covering the seven main areas of the programme. With each cartoon there is an explanation of the purpose of the underlying rationale of the material covered. The cartoon material in this programme sets out clearly, humorously and sympathetically what can often be sensitive areas, such as alcohol consumption or the role of the grandmother, as well as providing material across the whole spectrum of family health and development.

The programme

The child development programme is complex and wide-ranging and, at the risk of oversimplification, it may be useful to summarize nine of its unique and more important features:

(1)   The programme stresses the importance of working with the parents and recognizes that the parents are the experts of their own children.

(2)   There is a pattern of regular monthly visits made by appointment. The emphasis is on the health visitor sharing responsibility with the parents and eliciting a more in depth response than may be possible in a traditional visit.

(3)   There is a recognition that while the child is the focus of attention, the health and self-esteem of the mother is also of crucial importance.

(4)   The health visitor does not carry out ideas with the child herself, as this can make parents feel inadequate.

(5)   There is a positive approach towards the child's development and reasons are always found to praise something that the mother is doing.

(6)   There is an emphasis on the idea of child-rearing being a matter of enjoyment, a concept which is often missing in other programmes which emphasize precise goals, tasks and achievements, like some form of duty.

It may also be useful here to draw on material from the home visiting manual on these issues, so that some idea is gained about the approach that is recommended.

'Child-rearing a matter of joy and skill'
It will be hard to persuade many mothers that child rearing can be 'fun' – a combination of some skilled effort and much joy at the partial successes. This view should, however, motivate the health visitor's whole approach, if possible. Thus the demands that are implied when the mother simply opts out of everything.

The following are some suggested ways of dealing with particular (and important) problems:

(a) *A parent who 'does not have any time':* the mother could be asked to estimate, as a matter of interest to the visitor, how much time she actually spends interacting (playing, talking, washing, etc.) with the child each day and what periods of time are used for other activities; merely discussing the allocation of the hours, without the visitor offering any suggestions, may help to focus the mother's awareness.

(b) *On 'language interaction':* here again the importance of deliberately making time to *talk* to the infant can be stressed; one might suggest that the mother tries to estimate how much time she spends on necessary care of the child, e.g. on nappy changing, feeding, bathing, soothing. At least that time could be used for deliberate 'talk-play' – rhymes or other pleasant talk to the infant – aimed at fostering the child's language skills.

(c) *On 'how the child behaves':* the mother can be helped to understand that a great deal of the child's early social behaviour comes from its inborn temperament; while temperament cannot be blamed for every problem behaviour it is helpful for the mother to realize that the child's unique temperament contributes to how it is reacting to her and to others. A further point here is to help the mother realize that her response to that child's behaviours can in turn influence the development of later social behaviours; she will therefore need to learn that great care is needed to handle the behaviours tactfully.

(d) *On 'thinking':* it is often not realized that a child's mental abilities can be profoundly altered by the kinds of activities it is given – altered for the worse or for the better. At every age it is possible to think up simple puzzle activities or 'problem-solving' tasks which will stimulate the child's imagination and mental functioning. It is preferable to leave only a small number of educational or other toys with the child at any one time to foster the child's powers of concentration.

(e) *On 'education':* for every child the first and most important teacher is the mother, and the second most important is a helpful and interested partner. There is a great deal that parents can do to prepare the child for school, right from the first year. The parents can help particularly by showing the child picture books and talking about the pictures, by reading stories to the child every night before the child goes to sleep, by playing simple number games and by teaching the child how to manipulate objects, e.g. by sorting toys (into soft/hard or other divisions), clothing (sizes or who they belong to), and eating utensils.

(f) *On 'feeding the child':* here it is helpful to ask the mother what she thinks may be missing from the child's diet, or how she thinks it might be improved, rather than the health visitor giving her a more frank assessment. One cannot overstate the importance of the request to the mother to recall everything that her child ate the previous day. This arouses the mother's and visitor's interest in a typical diet. The judgment of that diet can be far more perceptive than when relying on a vague discussion about what the child eats. The programme under discussion has a variety of documentation available, including simple illustrated instructions, to help the health visitor obtain this nutritional information.

(g) *On 'health':* this field, including the questions of safety, is too well known to health visitors and other nurses to need any expansion in the present guides. What has been learned in this programme, however, is that suggestions about imperatives such as having a child immunized or putting a safety guard around the fire appear to be more acceptable if they are part of a total support package, rather than being the only purpose of a visit.

(7) The health visitor is encouraged not to let other non-developmental concerns take up more than one third of the time of the visit, except in cases of crisis. Other issues should be referred to the appropriate agency. This restriction of the content is quite an interesting feature in that clients themselves often bring up a wide range of issues for discussion in the traditional visit, but may do so only because they are not clear about the purpose of the visit in the first instance (Orr, 1980).

(8) There is a recognition that such intervention can be difficult in

particular circumstances. The visiting guide highlights these and gives the following guidance:

Particular problems

Among the serious problems which might arise during the support programme, most will be apparent to sensitive visitors and can be left to their sound common sense to handle, e.g. holding back the (very rare) mother who is too pushy towards her child, or observing and reporting non-accidental injury (NAI) cases, although it may well happen that the support programme itself reduces the likelihood of such incidents.

A few points need special mention:

(a)   *Mother–child bond.*

In situations where the emotional bonds between mother and child are extremely bad, or non-existent, it is likely to prove very difficult to conduct a satisfactory support programme, unless the visitor can find ways of strengthing the emotional bonds or at least helping the mother to recognize the difficulties caused by this situation; alternatively the main thrust of the support work could be focused on the father or other partner, provided that the mother agrees.

(b)   *Disadvantage.*

In situations of serious disadvantage a mother may passively accept whatever is suggested, without really believing in the strategies, and may fail to express her disagreement or doubts about particular proposals. Again it is important to persuade such mothers to express their doubts; these can then be examined and perhaps resolved with further support and encouragement from the visitor, or with modifications of the proposals to suit whatever the mother is willing to attempt.

(c)   *Lack of parental enthusiasm.*

In situations where a parent's response is to say that she already knows and does everything that is suggested, it can demand much of the visitor's patience to continue working with someone who appears to be blocking any ideas or suggestions. A health visitor needs first to examine her own strategy and approach towards the parent, and only if she is reasonably confident that she is not presenting herself as too much of an expert, to try even harder to draw out the mother's ideas about what she (the mother) thinks she could do to foster the child's development 'beyond what you (the mother) are already doing'.

(d)   *Lack of parental will.*
A mother's personality will influence the way she responds to the programme. Some mothers may find it hard to be as active as a health visitor might wish, and may agree to every suggestion but not do much. The health visitor will need to rethink her support methods and try to find activities which will arouse the mother's keenness. The uniqueness of every parent, mother or father, should always be recognized in the strategies used. Offering a uniform support programme to each family, or bringing in, say, the same set of cartoons to everyone, can seriously reduce the effectiveness of the programme.

(9)   Health visitors are provided with report forms for use at the ante-natal or primary visit and at each monthly visit. In addition, the parents are given a developmental card on which the health visitor records attainments each month.

Ante-natal and primary evaluation assessment

The ante-natal form focuses on how the health visitor can help the mother to plan for the future. Questions include whether the mother felt in control of what happened during the birth and whether her opinions about the management of the delivery were sought. The major areas covered are:

* Links with the surrounding community
* Housing
* Family environment
* Health environment
* Educational environment
* Mother's health – in particular the level of self-esteem and depression
* Life stresses such as who the mother can confide in.

In every case there is an immediate and sympathetic focus on what the parent can do to help improve a situation if problems are noted. Only if the parents' own resources are insufficient does the visitor offer further help. Again this is a way of supporting the parent rather than increasing her dependence.

Child progress report

The child progress report has two health sections, one for the recording of formal clinic/GP/hospital contacts and one for reporting on the health of the under 5s as seen and described by the mother. A brief note is made of everything the child (or children) ate or drank the previous day. Following sensitive and indirect questioning, note is made of the extent to which the tasks agreed at the previous month's visit have been carried out. The parent is asked specifically about what new ideas she (or he) has attempted in the previous month. Finally after extended discussion of possible goals for the month ahead, a note is made of what the parent plans to undertake and a copy of the mother's agreed goals is left with her as well.

A separate section at the end of the form is completed back in the clinic. This is a brief marking on the analogue scale, of the health visitor's assessment of:

(1)   The quality of the parent and home environment (as it affects the child) in seven areas of interest, i.e. health, nutrition, language, social, cognitive, early educational and emotional.
(2)   The level of development of the child (or children) in each of these same seven areas (see Appendix 6).

More recent developments

Two developments arising from the original model raise important issues for health visiting. An evaluation instrument known as the 'Early Health and Development Monitor' is now being used in nearly half of the 25 health authorities collaborating in the Child Development Programme. This instrument has a twofold purpose: to assess the effectiveness of programme visiting in line with the unit's belief that whatever is done should be subjected to ongoing monitoring; and to provide regular reports on the most significant outcomes of health visiting in relation to the health and development of young children throughout the health authority.

The monitor is used to gather a modest amount of information during a 20-minute monitor visit to the home each year; this information is recorded on a single card which covers the first four years of a child's life, and the card is immediately sent in to the authority's central office for data input on to a hard disk micro-computer. The focus in the monitor's development has been on creating something which is relatively informal in appearance and yet fairly rigorous in the way it has to be completed. By making use of micro-computers the unit avoids the complexities of trying to persuade the authority's mainframe computers to produce usable and localized information at the touch of a button – something which can be done on micros programmed for the monitor.

It is worth noting that although the instrument was initially devised purely as a field tool for evaluating Child Development Programme effectiveness, its primary function today is to offer health authorities, epidemiologists and others, and not least health visitors and their managers, an easily analysable packet of information on health outcomes at any level, ranging from across the authority down to individual caseloads.

What this instrument is saying is that health visiting, at least as far as the under-fives and their parents are concerned, is accountable and measurable as outcomes. It is a sharp contrast to the Korner philosophy which motivates much information input in the health service today, namely the measurement of activity, regardless of how effective or otherwise that activity may be. For health visitors and their managers the monitor poses the choice of investing valuable time on gathering usable, interesting and potentially powerful information to justify health visiting itself, or not using the monitor and spending the time on other activities which may have a higher profile but are not necessarily convincing, as they have no measurable health outcomes.

A more contentious recent development has been the introduction of women with children living in the community to acts as community mothers, these women make home visits to selected families and make use of the same cartoons as do trained health visitors within the Child Development Programme. They also use simplified visiting forms. The women are selected on the basis of being experienced and competent mothers, who have the ability to empathize with and empower others. It is also a condition that they have to be living on the same housing estates as the families they visit. The first community mothers programme was set up by the Early Childhood Development Unit in Dublin six years ago. The community mothers are guided and trained by public health nurses. There are now 150 of them, visiting about 1000 first-time families a year. The movement is strong and growing, and has - after a stormy birth - received the enthusiastic approval of the Irish-Nurses' Organization.

Recently, modified versions of this same programme have been initiated in the UK within two communities. In one city an Asian Parent Programme has been initiated, using Asian women from within specific Pakistani or Indian immigrant communities, to do home visits using cartoons translated (and modified where necessary) into Urdu or Gujarati.

An equally interesting development has been the initiation of a community mothers programme in a socially stressed area on the south-east coast. It is an area where first-parent visiting is already being undertaken. The community mothers work with multiple families referred to them by the generic visitor colleagues of the first-parent visitors; the families are selected on the grounds of their social and child-rearing problems. As the community mothers come from the same neighbourhood as the families they visit, they have a street credibility which no professional could equal.

The unit's development of the last-named programme, and of some other community mother programmes which are now under considera-tion in the UK, poses major questions about the health visiting role at a time when skill mix is a concept being introduced in many authorities. The unit's contention (personal communication) is that community mothers, who almost by definition lack any formal health qualifications, cannot be seen as a replacement for the professional role of health visitors.

Clearly, this study is already having an impact on health visiting. Its approach to parents highlights what are often little explored areas in the relationship between clients and health visitors. We will now move on to look at other issues in the health visitor and client relationship.

HEALTH VISITOR/CLIENT RELATIONSHIP

The health visitor/client relationship is significant in that it is utilized in order to collect data, identify problems, formulate a plan and set both short-term and long-term goals with the client's assistance. The relation-ship is a therapeutic vehicle in the giving of care and advice as it enables the health visitor and client to move through the orientation, working and termination stages of the problem-solving process. It will be characterized by both growth and regression, but can be said to be significant since it is 'a mutual learning experience' (Stuart & Sundeen, 1979) and it is essential for the health visitor and the client to become partners in the problem-solving process. It is a situation in which those involved are 'in the process of becoming'. Within a relationship there is respect for different values and the uniqueness of each individual is observed and respected. If such a relationship exists, the health visitor cannot force anything on the client but must recognize that often the client will have different standards which must be respected and observed.

The relationship is seen to be a therapeutic one and as such is the vehicle for employing strategies which will lead to the achievement of defined goals, facilitating the feeling of trust between the health visitor and client. Trust is defined as 'the connection with one another, and to have a firm belief in each other's honesty, reliability and accountability'

(Wiedenback & Falls, 1978). Trust is the foundation upon which effective practice is built, and it is a necessary part of the relationship if health visitors and clients are to work together and follow a problem-solving process. It is the therapeutic relationship that facilitates the growth and strengthens the trust between health visitor and client.

The health visitor cannot remain outside or separate from the relationship with the individual client. The relationship is not a static entity nor does it have clearly defined boundaries. There are contradictions, ambiguities and conflicts within the relationship and roles are constantly being renegotiated. The interaction has the features of any one to one relationship: it is affected by both participants and both participants are affected by it. This type of relationship has two elements, the observed and the observer, the known and the unknown, but it is in the very act of observing that the observer becomes the observed and the unknown the known. The fluidity of the interaction belies the traditional image of the client/professional relationship in which the professional conducts an interview without deviating from the aims, being side-tracked by the client or being asked direct questions about their personal life. There is an assumption that the client will act in a way which is acceptable and to ensure this, professionals have an investment in defining the way things are (Becker, 1967). This definition is reflected in the kind of services offered, whom they are offered to and by the methods of service delivery employed. In essence, the professional's concept of the client's problems shapes what the professional believes is needed. The reason for this is that, within a fairly limited perspective, professionals define client needs by professional skills. If we, as professionals, cannot resolve or come to terms with problems then these problems will not be recognized. Cases of child abuse, abused women and incest are examples of problems which were little recognized because society had few solutions to offer in the context of their being social problems.

But what about the interaction from the client's perspective? The very nature of the visit from the health visitor must appear to the client to have some of the characteristics of any other visit by a friend or relative. There are, of course, differences which are apparent, such as the health visitor being the one to initiate the visit, determine its length and have some purpose in calling. In addition, the client is aware that the health visitor has information of a personal nature relating to the family and has some power over the fate of the family. The interaction, despite this, may be perceived by the client to be similar to any conversation in which she is at liberty to ask questions in order to establish who the health visitor is and what type of person she is. There is no doubt that the health visitor is being observed and judgments are being made as to her attitudes, friendliness, knowledge and personal appearance. At some point the client realizes that this is more than a normal type of social visit and may at that stage become concerned as to her role and appropriate conduct. After all the client has not had intensive training on how to be a client, and may not even recognize the label 'client'. This label is given by the professional, of course, to distinguish the differences in status and training. The client may not accept the idea of being dependent on professional help and may have considerable confidence in being a mother. We can see her as a professional mother by dint of experience.

We define ourselves largely by the jobs we do and this applies no less to mothers than to health visitors. Just as professionals place emphasis on their particular skills and role so mothers also need to have their skills and efforts recognized and valued. If we accept that complex skills are needed for even simple tasks we need appreciate the complexity of mothering, which at the very least requires intelligence, imagination, determination, humour, patience and strength.

The client may exhibit considerable skills in defending her integrity and may be accomplished in manipulating the interaction. As health visitors, we are aware of the social skills which are used in an interaction and the difficulties of employing such skills as listening or questioning. Yet we do not seem to recognize the efforts of the client in listening and the emotional labouring it takes to reflect on feelings or discuss emotive issues. How often do we recognize that a visit may be tiring for the client as well as for us and that the client may be expending considerable energy in hosting the visit? In the context of health visiting Chalmers and Luker (1991) have provided an in-depth examination of the issues involved in building and maintaining the relationship.

The health visitor has to recognize that she may impose her reality on the visit. We may see what we want to see, or what we have been taught to expect. How do we identify what is and what is known? As health visitors, our knowledge comes from our own experiences and our training; however, there is no guarantee that the subjects we study fully describe the reality of people's lives and often it is the experiences of women that have been discounted and devalued. This is important for health visitors in that their work is largely with women (Dunnell & Dobbs, 1983). Science and social science tend to serve to reinforce dominant social values and conceptions of reality as much as, and often more than, they serve to challenge them. There is as yet no psychology of women, no sociology of women, no anthropology of women, no real history of women and no thorough and coherent social science theory about women (Du Bois, 1983). In fact, until recently, sociology was a male science of society, and has been a sociology of the male world (Bernard, 1973). The problems and priorities of women were regarded as less important and where women did come into sociology it was as they related to men and the problems they posed for them.

The exclusion of women extends from the classification of subject areas and definition of topics and methods of empirical research, to the construction of models and theories (Oakley, 1974). It is only through sociologists like Oakley that main areas of women's lives such as housework, childbirth and child-rearing have been explored and investigated (Oakley, 1980). This increasing body of knowledge has crucial relevance for health visitors both in their work with women and in their own lives as women. Of particular importance is the work on language which is analysed by Spender (1980). A description is given by Spender of how language is created by men and how the male is seen as the norm and the female as deviating from that norm. She also argues that there are few words which adequately describe many women's experiences.

Spender has highlighted the 'inaudibility' of women in the case of motherhood, and this is relevant to health visitors. According to Spender motherhood in our society has a legitimated meaning which is equated with 'feminine fulfilment, and which leaves women consumed and replete with joy.' While it is the case that motherhood can have this meaning for some women, Spender argues that it is only a partial meaning and that it is false to portray this as the only meaning. Health visitors are aware that motherhood may have been a different and traumatic experience for many mothers, but because these mothers cannot relate to the legitimated meaning they are left feeling inadequate, estranged and isolated. There is no adequate space within the meaning of the word motherhood to accommodate their experience. If this is the case for the word 'motherhood' it is possible that other meanings are also inadequate. The work of Oakley and other feminists raises questions for health visitors about how much they should be involved in helping women validate their experiences, as opposed to helping to perpetuate essentially male values and meanings.

CONCLUSION

The development of the State's responsibility for child-bearing, child-rearing and health care reflects the change from the laissez-faire liberalism of the past to the highly developed social welfare services of modern Britain. Health visitors and community workers have played a part in these changes and have been influenced by them; the health visitor, for example, acts as a link between the family and the State and is confronted by the lack of consensus between societal need and resources. Health visitors operate uneasily on the interface between what appears unlimited need and very limited and shrinking resources. There is a requirement to see the issues surrounding intervention in families as essentially political. When, for example, health visitors express concern about families and describe the strains imposed by poverty or poor housing they are identifying a reality which is political in terms of access to scarce resources and hence they are suggesting political and economic solutions to individual problems. Here, we have addressed issues surrounding the concept of need and have attempted to present a critical examination of the relationship between the health visitor and the family. There are ways through which health visitors can develop their work with families, and it is hoped that the approaches we have suggested will go some way towards providing a more critical and challenging service.

5   Evaluating Practice

Karen Luker

EVALUATION IN HEALTH CARE

Evaluation as a component of the nursing process is examined in the general context of nursing and in the particular area of community health nursing. Health care has been described by Karhausen (1978) as 'the set of actions which aim at the improvement of individual and collective health levels'. Health care can be seen to be the concern of a number of professional groups including health visitors.

In recent years other groups of nurses working in the community have extended their own knowledge base to include work which was traditionally thought of as health visiting. Given that roles are evolving but titles are not yet changing, we have tended to use the traditional term health visiting here.

The greater emphasis now placed on the evaluation of health care services stems from the escalating costs brought about by the increased complexity of the service and the decreasing purchasing power of the pound. The increased complexity of the service has been caused by medical and technical advances and has resulted in a proliferation of the numbers of paramedical staff. Moreover, the increase in paramedical staff has influenced the practice of other professional groups, most notably nurses. The increasing trend towards specialization initiated by medicine and mirrored in nursing has resulted in greater competition for limited resources. The uncertainty generated by the fact that demand exceeds supply, in terms of finance, has meant that doctors and nurses alike are forced to look for verifiable facts to assist them in establishing a convincing case worthy of continued or additional financial support. Reid and Holland (1978) state that 'until now, the majority of policy decisions in the health care field have simply followed a logical appraisal of the options and people involved in decision-making.' Thus, current decision-making which may result in the expenditure of large amounts of public money is commonly based on the past experience of a collection of individuals and not on pertinent, factual data. In order to justify society's continued support and commitment to health care it is necessary to provide 'proof' of effectiveness (Suchman, 1967). The 1990 National Health Service and Social Care Act has placed evaluation firmly on every professional's agenda. Such evaluation was previously an optional extra; it now has to become an essential ingredient if services are to continue at present or increased levels and be responsive to change.

Evaluation – the problem of definition

The word 'evaluation' is widely used and for the most part its meaning is taken for granted. Few attempts have been made to formulate a conceptually rigorous definition of evaluation or to analyse the meanings behind its use. The lack of a clear definition has meant that the word 'evaluation' is used interchangeably with other terms such as 'assessment' and 'appraisal'. We talk of assessment or evaluation in the context of client or community needs and indeed assessment is said to be the first stage in the nursing process and evaluation the last. We hear nurse managers talk of staff appraisal or evaluation and this relates to how well individual practitioners are functioning in their particular role. It is evident then that confusion may arise if we use the word evaluation in a casual way.

Taking into account the common usage of the term evaluation Suchman (1967) makes the distinction between 'evaluation' and 'evaluative research'. Evaluation when used in a general way is said to refer to the everyday occurrence of making judgments of worth. Although this interpretation implies some form of logical or rational thought it does not presuppose any systematic procedures for presenting objective evidence to support the judgment. Evaluation when used in this way refers only to the process of assessment or appraisal of worth. Evaluative research on the other hand implies the utilization of scientific methods and techniques for the purpose of making an evaluation. Inherent in the terms evaluative research is an emphasis on the measurement of change. Riecken (1952) defines evaluation as 'The measurement of desirable and undesirable consequences of an action that has been taken in order to forward some goal that we value'. The distinction that Suchman (1967) makes between evaluation and evaluative research may seem irrelevant or daunting to some practitioners who consider that they will never become involved in research as a primary activity. However, what Suchman is suggesting is that a distinction should be made between unsubstantiated judgments of worth and substantiated judgments of worth. In our everyday work as community health nurses we are constantly involved in making judgments of worth. For example, if we simply say that we believe that visits to the elderly are a good idea this is an unsubstantiated judgment. If on the other hand we say that visits to the elderly are good because they reduce the incidence of loneliness and depression amongst this age group then this is a substantiated judgment. If we have some insight into the criteria used as the basis of the statement this does not make it research but it does imply that we have some evidence to support our position. Other community health nurses may not agree with our criteria but this is not essential. During the past five years a great deal has been written about evaluation; the impetus has come from the desire to measure the effectiveness or adequacy of care. (Alderman, 1989; Hull, 1989; McCall, 1988). Despite the upsurge of interest in the topic theoretically, nothing new has emerged. There has in the main been a revisiting of old issues and themes.

In conceptualizing the various approaches to evaluation the goal attainment model stands out as being particularly appealing to those involved in the evaluation of health care. The notion of goal attainment is embodied in the target setting approach adopted by many health authorities; a good example of this are the immunization and cervical screening targets set by FHSAs.

Schulberg and Baker (1968) acknowledge that there is popular agreement amongst those concerned with evaluation that the most important and yet most difficult phase of the process is the clarification of objectives. The emphasis on objectives or goals stems from a conceptualization of evaluation as measurement of the success or failure of an activity in so far as it reaches its predetermined objectives.

The process of evaluating can be complex and it is always subjective. Evaluation involves a combination of basic assumptions underlying the activity to be evaluated and the personal values of those engaged in the activities being evaluated. Hence the process of evaluation always starts with a recognition of values and these values may be either explicit or implicit. In the context of health visiting, Robinson (1985) provides a useful insight into the difficulties involved in attaching meaning to the values which underpin practice such as 'health'. Furthermore, the complexities involved in defining health as either individual or collective are explored. Despite evaluation being problematic in the field of community health nursing, the evaluation process as described by Suchman (1967) is a useful starting point; this is represented with slight modification in Figure 5.1.

Example: slimming club

With reference to the evaluation process (Fig. 5.1), we will explore possible ways of evaluating a health programme. Let us suppose that we

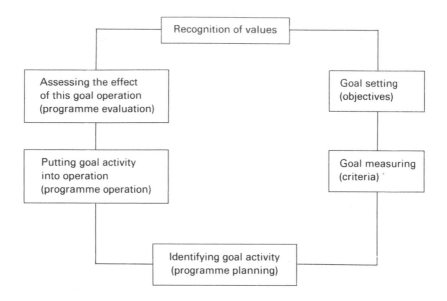

Fig. 5.1. The evaluation progress. From: Suchman, Edward A. (1967) *Evaluative Research: Principles and Practice in Public Service and Social Action Programs*, Russell Sage Foundation. Reprinted by permission of the publishers, Basic Books, New York.

are community health nurses responsible for health education in a comprehensive school. We have observed that there appear to be a large number of overweight children in the classes we teach. Our observations will reflect our values. Firstly, we believe that to be overweight in adolescence is bad; we may also hold different views on why this is undesirable. Some of us may believe that overweight adolescents experience more upper respiratory tract infections and may be more prone to develop coronary artery disease in later life. Others may be of the opinion that fat adolescents do not look as attractive as those of average or light build and this may lead to an internalization of a negative self-image. In part these value judgments reflect the beliefs and values of the society in which we live and work. In response to this perceived need we decide to set up a slimming club. The underlying rationale of this action is that we believe that it would be beneficial to the individuals concerned to lose weight and furthermore we believe it would benefit society if the next generation of parents were fit and healthy.

The objectives of the slimming club will probably be wider than just getting the children to lose weight, although this will, of course, be the major focus. Firstly we may have to convince the overweight adolescents that to be obese is undesirable and a potential threat to future health and wellbeing. But this approach presupposes that they will place a value on health; we may instead have to appeal to their vanity and suggest that they may look more attractive if they were slimmer. As community health nurses we see ourselves as health educators and it is likely that we will use the slimming club to teach the children about the nutritional value of food and the value of a balanced diet. There is scope for individual practitioners to think of additional objectives which may be more or less important than those already stated. After identifying our objectives or goals the next stage of the evaluation process is to clarify how we will determine when the goal has been achieved. Looking back at our objectives, we can identify a number of possible criteria on which we will base our judgment concerning the success or failure of the slimming club.

Firstly, the number of children who attend the club and the frequency of their attendance. This may give us some indication as to whether the club was seen as useful by the children. However, we have to be careful how we interpret these data because whether children attend the club or not depends to some extent on structural factors and we will come back to this topic when thinking about programme planning.

Secondly, unlike most areas of community health nursing in this context we are fortunate in having one truly objective criteria and that is the amount of weight that each child actually loses. In addition, once a child has attained his or her target weight then we would expect the weight to remain constant and not continue to fall. It goes almost without saying that in order to measure weight accurately we need a reliable pair of scales and the children should be weighed in the same or similar clothes each week.

Thirdly, given that our objectives suggest that we want the children to understand something about the nutritional value of food, it may therefore be useful to compare what the children knew before they attended the slimming club with what they know after they have been exposed to lectures and other teaching sessions on the nutritional value of food. This data or information may best be obtained by giving the children a questionnaire to fill in on the first visit to the club and then a follow-up questionnaire after the sessions on nutrition. This would give us some indication of their knowledge level and some feedback as to whether or not our teaching sessions have been successful.

In order to achieve our goals the evaluation process suggests that we devise a strategy for setting up our slimming club. First it would be helpful to know how many children would be interested in coming to a slimming club. We could find out this information by putting a poster in each of the classrooms inviting children who consider themselves to be overweight to attend a meeting either at lunchtime or immediately after school. Given that there is some interest at the subsequent meeting, discussion could take place about the time and location for the proposed slimming club meetings (obviously if the meetings are held at inconvenient times and places then attendance will be poor). The next step is to decide how the club will be run. Will there, for example, be a health education input every week? Will other health professionals be asked to take part such as the dietitian or physiotherapist? Will there be an exercise session? Once this is done we then have to meet the challenge of putting the programme into action.

We may find that in the early stages we need to make modifications. For example, we may find that is is better to put the formal lecture before rather than after the exercise session; perhaps it will be necessary to enlist the support of some colleagues and do more group work. There are always teething problems when launching any new programme and time is well spent in the early stages making adjustments and modifications. Once the programme is well established we begin to think more carefully about the final stage of the evaluation process, i.e. judging the effects of the programme. It is important to remember that it is usual to evaluate a programme in terms of its goals and the goal measuring criteria are the key to the evaluation. In addition we may wish to collect supplementary information which might help us with future planning. We could, for exmaple, encourage the consumers to suggest ways in which we could improve the slimming club. Our evaluation, that is our judgment about whether or not the club was a success or failure, feeds back into our value system and the whole process is repeated.

Example: Well Women Clinic

When offering a different kind of service to meet the perceived needs of a particular group in the current economic climate, there is an imperative to evaluate the effect of the innovation in order to justify a continuation of the service or to gain additional resources. The Manchester Well Women Clinic is an example of an innovation in health care that was evaluated. The Well Women Clinic was set up in a deprived area of the city, the intention of the health district was that the clinic should be viewed only as a pilot scheme. Spencer *et al.* defined the main target group for the clinic as 'women who rarely if ever visit their doctor and who are believed medically to be most at risk, i.e. the disadvantaged, the poor, the infertile and the older women' (Spencer *et al.*, 1982). They also saw the goals or aims of the Well Women Clinic as threefold:

(1) To reach women who usually avoid visiting the doctor for reasons of class, culture or sex of the doctor
(2) To attempt to discover effective ways of meeting women's specific health needs
(3) To develop insight into the problems involved in providing health care to this group, so that the services and information which contribute to good health care of the individual and the community can be offered in an acceptable form.

As the clinic was set up as a pilot scheme, plans were made for a formal evaluation to take place. With this in view, first-time attenders were asked to complete a questionnaire which, when put together with the results of certain screening procedures, were said to constitute a 'health profile'. A copy of this was kept by both the women and the clinic and this was used to formulate health promotion proposals for each attender. The evaluation of the clinic has been made mainly on the basis of the information contained in the health profile. In brief, the findings indicate that the clinic fulfilled the aims it set out to achieve. The women who attended the clinic were found to have large numbers of health problems of physical, psychological and social origins. The clinic was used mainly by older women and few used the clinic simply for screening or a check-up. It seemed that all attenders welcomed the opportunity to take advantage of the facilities offered and most enjoyed being able to talk over their problems in a relaxed atmosphere. Most notable was the incidence of gynaecological problems amongst these women. A high number of referrals were made following vaginal examinations where over half the women were found to have a vaginal discharge or other gynaecological symptoms. In fact gynaecological symptoms were often instrumental in bringing the women to the clinic in the first place. It would seem that women may be reluctant to take their female complaints to their family doctor and may shy away from visiting special clinics. Hence these gynaecological problems are often dealt with by the cytology screening services since women use the facilities intended for population screening as a diagnostic service. According to Spencer *et al.* (1982) this is an inefficient use of scarce resources. The incidence of gynaecological disorders in the women who attended the Manchester clinic points up a gap in current services and on the basis of the data collected in this pilot study it would seem that Well Women Clinics could be one effective solution to this problem. This evaluation of the Well Women Clinic has provided the innovators or programme planners with some factual evidence on which they can base a case for continued and additional financial support. In terms of financial cutbacks in the health service it is no longer sufficient to say that we believe a service to be effective; we have to demonstrate, in unequivocal terms, that it is.

THE NURSING PROCESS

It would appear that the goal attainment approach towards evaluation is applicable to community health nursing at an individual and family level since goal setting and evaluation are operationalized through the nursing process. The nursing process is fundamentally a problem-solving approach to care and this has a tendency to make it appear alien to traditional health visitors since they perceive it as diminishing their preventive function. In the context of health visiting a proposition discussed by Robinson (1982) is that the different theoretical perspectives taught during health visitor training suggest two possible models of practice. The first model is founded on a clinical problem-orientated base and it is claimed that the theoretical underpinnings of this approach are found in basic nurse and midwifery training. The second model suggested by Robinson is founded on a relationship-centred base and it is claimed that the theoretical underpinnings may be found in the teaching of social science. Within this approach the clients engage in the identification of factors affecting their health and wellbeing. It would seem that the two models suggested by Robinson are too simplistic to provide an adequate account of health visiting practice. It would appear that a nursing process approach can transcend both Robinson's models and keep in perspective the preventive function of community health nursing by focusing on actual and potential health problems of individuals and age cohorts (Mayers, 1972).

Actual and potential problems

In the past, health visitors were reluctant to consider themselves involved in dealing with clients' health problems. Instead they have reiterated their uniqueness in so far as they claim to visit families many of whom have no apparent health problems. Although this may be true for a small minority of families in terms of actual health problems, intuitively it cannot be the case in the context of potential problems. The word 'problem' is often associated by many health visitors with that nebulous term 'problem family'. However, in this context, a health problem is defined as a matter which concerns the health visitor or client about the client's health at the time of the visit or assessment. Actual problems are those which are present at the time of the assessment or follow-up visit. Potential problems are not present; instead there are indicators or cues which suggest that an actual problem may develop if no action is taken. it is feasible that with the expansion of the role of other nurses working in the community to include preventive health care, that similar difficulties may be voiced when discussing problem identification. Nevertheless, it is suggested that the notion of actual and potential problems is broad enough to relate to the work of all community health nurses.

An example of an actual problem at an assessment visit may be that of a baby with a sore eye, a baby who refuses to suck at the breast, or a child who has regressed to soiling himself. Health visitors are more concerned with potential problems, i.e. preventing actual problems occurring. An example of a potential problem for a couple expecting a baby who already have a two-year-old child might be jealousy on the part of the toddler after the baby is born. The health visitor would be keen to assist the parents in preventing this problem occurring. She would, therefore, discuss ways in which the family might begin to prepare the two-year-old for the birth of the new baby. Discussion may also follow concerning the management of the toddler during his first separation from his mother which is, of course, inevitable if the birth is to take place in hospital. By intervening before there is an actual problem the health visitor tries to promote the wellbeing of the whole family. Since health visitor clients are not put through any test of eligibility this means that some clients will have no actual health problems but almost all will have at least one potential health problem; this is not the case for clients visited, for example, by a district nurse.

Community health nurses visit families from conception to the grave. If we view life as a developmental time span then theoretically it can be argued that the younger one is, the more potential health problems one has and the fewer actual problems. Conversely, the older one is, the more actual problems one experiences and the relative risk of potential problems developing is reduced. However, a potential problem is usually only considered by the practitioner if it has a higher than average probability of becoming an actual problem. For example, all babies are at risk of developing obesity; the infant whose siblings or parents are obese, however, would be considered by the community health nurse to have a potential problem in this area. Similarly, all elderly people could be said to be at risk from falling. However, this may only be recorded as a potential problem if there were factors present which suggested that there was an above average risk of the client falling. For example, if the elderly person had failing vision due to senile cataracts or dizzy spells as a result of Menière's disease or had been reported to have had previous falls then the client may be deemed to have a potential problem in this area.

Problem-solving

The nursing process is made up of a number of components:

(1) Data collection
(2) Goal setting
(3) Care planning
(4) Intervention
(5) Evaluation

Other analogous terms may be found in the literature on the nursing process. It is noteworthy that problem-solving is subjective and value

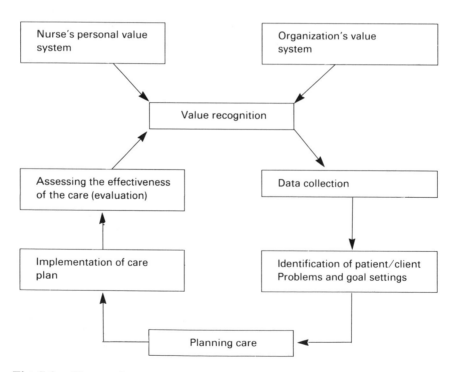

Fig. 5.2. The nursing process.

laden in so far as nurses and health visitors collect data and identify problems which they or the recipients of their care consider to be important. Hence the nursing process, like the evaluative process, begins with a recognition of values (Fig. 5.2).

EVALUATION AND EVALUATIVE RESEARCH

Although the evaluation component of the nursing process is able to substantiate its claims, there are two reasons why it cannot be said to constitute evaluative research.

Firstly, in evaluative research the main thrust of the activity is directed towards measuring how far intervention has achieved or not achieved its goals whereas in the nursing process the measurement of the effectiveness of nursing care is subsidiary to the primary goal of giving care. Owing to the secondary purpose of evaluation in the nursing process goal statements may not be recorded; however, nurses are involved in making judgments of worth about the care which they give whether they record it or not. Many of these value judgments will be made on the basis of systematically collected data and experience, and, the evaluation criteria may vary between individuals.

Secondly, in evaluative research, data are collected on a predetermined target population and therefore findings may be related to more than one individual, whereas in the evaluative component of the nursing process the nurse evaluates the care she gives to each individual and is not in a position to determine her patients/clients in the same way as a researcher determines the sample.

All in all, evaluation may best be viewed as a continuum (Fig. 5.3). The

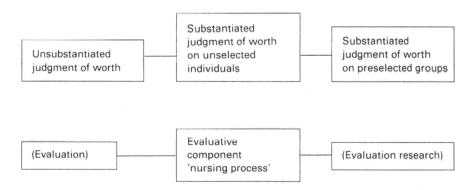

Fig. 5.3. Continuum of evaluation.

evaluation component of the nursing process can be placed almost anywhere along this continuum depending upon the way the data are collected (systematically or otherwise) and recorded. Data which have been systematically collected and recorded during the execution of the nursing process may be used retrospectively by nurses for research purposes. The retrospective use of the material may be referred to as 'evaluative research' because evaluation and not care giving has become the main thrust of the activity and the researcher is able to determine the population to be studied.

Evaluation of nursing care

Concern for the measurement of the quality of nursing care provided to patients/clients and attempts at evaluating care are not new. However, the desire to develop measurements of quality are possibly a relatively recent development in nursing. It may be possible to get agreement on the importance of evaluation. There is less agreement, however, about what will be evaluated and how the evaluation should be done (Hagen, 1972).

The North American literature on evaluation dates back to Derryberry (1939) who, in a report concerning the accomplishments of nursing, stated:

> 'in the past, evaluation of nursing services have been based upon volume and intensity of service . . . Evidence of the more elusive quality of service as expressed by the changing state of the patient has been sought in the present analysis.'

It is interesting that more than fifty years have passed since Derryberry made this plea to move away from evaluations based on volume and intensity of service in favour of focusing on patient/client outcome. However, within the context of community health nursing we have unfortunately failed to move very far forward.

The data most commonly used to provide insight into the work of, for example, health visitors at both a national and local level are the statistical data which relate to frequency of health visitor visits to particular client groups. It is possible for these statistics to be used to demonstrate how health visitors spend some of their time and this information may be useful to managers and policy makers. At a national level Table 5.1 gives some indication of the way health visitors spend their time between various client groups; this data also exists for each health district and for the district nursing service.

Issues concerning the allocation of resources and the establishment of priorities in health visiting have concerned nurse managers for some time. In an attempt to contribute to the resolution of these 'allocation problems' Wiseman (1979) has developed a model to assist in the attainment of health sector targets regarding health visitor visiting rates to various care groups. Wiseman's approach provides us with more information about who health visitors visit than that currently provided by government statistics. Undoubtedly the information generated by this case group approach is immensely valuable to the health district concerned. Nevertheless it must be said that statistics do not provide information about the outcome of health visitor visits to particular client groups. Currently, there is probably a consensus amongst community health nurses that care should be evaluated by means other than volume and intensity of service. Three major factors which are related to the type of care an individual receives have been highlighted by Lindeman (1976a; 1976b) and these are:

(1)   The setting in which the care is given
(2)   The actual care given
(3)   The outcome of care.

The decision to measure any of the factors which influence care will to some extent reflect values, beliefs and assumptions held about nursing. Hence the first step in evaluation has been described in Lindeman as conceptualization and this is in tune with Suchman (1967; Fig. 5.1) who stressed the importance of values being made explicit in any attempt at evaluation.

Structure, process and outcome evaluation

In the context of medical care evaluation, Donabedian (1969), a pioneer in this field, described three approaches to evaluation, i.e. structure evaluation, process evaluation and outcome evaluation. Donabedian's approach to evaluation corresponds to Lindeman's although the terminology used is different.

Structure evaluation

Structure evaluation involves the study of factors in the organization system, the availability of facilities and equipment, staffing levels, styles of management and the characteristics of the care givers. The assumption underlying this approach to evaluation is that if the facilities, staff

Table 5.1. Community health services: health and tuberculosis visitor services (DOH Health & Personal Social Services Statistics for England 1990.) (Reproduced by kind permission of Her Majesty's Stationery Office.)

England

	Unit	1978	1982	1983	1984	1985	1986	1987/88[1]	1988/89
Persons visited at home[2]									
Total	**Thousands**	**3,596.7**	**3,811.6**	**3,857.7**	**3,986.8**	**4,080.2**	**4,129.4**	**4,093.0**	..
Age:									
Born that year		605.4	632.7	638.0	645.3	658.8	671.4	730.6	..
Other children under 5		1,654.3	1,667.8	1,677.2	1,672.6	1,672.1	1,677.2	1,573.2	..
5-16		198.2	212.5	205.7	212.2	206.9	211.8	192.9	..
17-64		634.2	840.4	890.6	1,005.2	1,076.9	1,135.4	1,200.4	..
65 and over		504.6	458.2	446.3	451.6	465.5	433.6	395.9	..
Persons visited as a percentage of:	*Per cent*								
Total population[2]		*7.8*	*8.1*	*8.2*	*8.5*	*8.7*	*8.8*	*8.6*	..
Live births that year		*108.0*	*107.4*	*107.6*	*107.5*	*106.4*	*108.4*	*113.6*	..
Population 1-4		*73.5*	*72.3*	*71.2*	*70.7*	*70.8*	*71.0*	*65.1*	..
Population 5-16		*2.3*	*2.7*	*2.7*	*2.8*	*2.8*	*2.5*	*2.7*	..
Population 17-64		*2.3*	*2.9*	*3.1*	*3.4*	*3.6*	*3.7*	*4.0*	..
Population 65 and over		*7.4*	*6.4*	*6.3*	*6.4*	*6.5*	*6.0*	*5.3*	..
Total visits	**Thousands**								
Total		..	**12,806.0**	**12,957.9**	**13,360.4**	**13,516.7**	**13,548.4**	**13,384.4**	..
Age:									
Born that year		..	3,058.2	3,066.0	3,108.1	3,156.5	3,177.0	3,299.8	..
Other children under 5		..	5,355.4	5,376.1	5,391.6	5,344.5	5,267.1	4,944.3	..
5-16		..	488.6	475.2	502.5	481.9	492.6	451.6	..
17-64		..	2,535.9	2,719.6	3,067.0	3,300.7	3,479.1	3,637.0	..
65 and over		..	1,367.9	1,321.0	1,291.2	1,233.1	1,132.7	1,051.7	..

Visited at home[2] included above (Thousands)								
Mentally handicapped persons	19.4	17.7	18.6	18.5	19.5	19.1	17.3	..
Mentally ill persons	23.4	15.1	14.5	13.8	14.6	13.6	14.1	..
Total visits to: (Thousands)								
Mentally handicapped persons	..	68.8	74.5	76.3	80.7	79.6	66.9	..
Mentally ill persons	..	63.3	57.3	55.2	54.8	52.7	49.4	..
Households visited on account of: (Thousands)								
Tuberculosis	37.0	29.4	24.2	21.4	21.3	21.0	18.0	..
Other infectious diseases	17.1	13.4	13.6	16.4	15.8	15.0	16.0	..
Total visits on account of: (Thousands)								
Tuberculosis	..	84.4	70.9	68.4	64.3	56.9	52.5	..
Other infectious diseases	..	30.7	28.7	31.1	30.1	27.9	32.2	..
Staff[3] (Wte)								
Health visitors[4]	7,807	9,350	9,550	9,214	10,147	10,353	10,293	10,276
Health visitor students	898	1,069	1,023	971	866	832	785	786
Tuberculosis visitors[5]	104	55	50	45	45	48	45	36

1 From 1987 collection of data changed from years ended 31 December to years ended 31 March.

2 Each person is counted at the first visit in the year in a district, by any member of the health visiting staff. A person moving to a new district will be counted more than once.

3 At 30 September.

4 Includes health visitor field work teachers, TB visitors with HV certificate, HV/DN/midwives and bank health visitors; excludes school health visitors. Due to changes in definition, figures for years prior to 1980 are not comparable with those for later years.

5 Without health visitor certificate.

and equipment reach specified standards then the care which follows will be 'good' and patients/clients will benefit. In keeping with this approach it would be assumed that health districts who have achieved their health visitor client ratio target of, for example, one health visitor per 2500 of the population should be providing a 'better' service than districts which fall below this target level.

Clearly skill-mix is a topical issue in community health nursing. We have grown accustomed to the notion of nurses trained to work in a particular speciality, e.g. traditionally health visiting and district nursing. The demographic changes, that is growing numbers of elderly people and fewer school leavers, coupled with the economic imperative, have forced us to re-think how best to use resources. We therefore expect to see more health care assistants and post Project 2000 nurses working in the community in the not-too-distant future.

Process evaluation

Process evaluation focuses on the staff which give the care to patients/clients in terms of whether or not the care was appropriate and carried out in the correct manner. The emphasis is firmly on what the nurse does and may also include decision-making. This may be considered as the traditional or taken-for-granted approach to evaluation.

If we ask community health nurses about the effects of their work they usually begin by telling us what they do. Hence the success of the visit is measured in terms of whether the nurse has achieved what she set out to do. For example, did she successfully complete an elderly person's health assessment or carry out a developmental assessment on a one-year-old child? The emphasis is on what the nurse has done and this can be partially accounted for by reflecting on the type of information that community health nurses are required to keep. Monthly or weekly statistical returns are filled in by all community nurses. Although the forms may vary from district to district it commonly instructs the nurse to record the initial purpose of the visit and the age group or care category of the client. The statistics collected in this way are collated centrally and used to demonstrate the range and volume of work done by health visitors and other community staff such as district nurses (see Table 5.1).

The report of Working Group D of the Steering Group on Health Services Information on Community Health Services Information was chaired by Edith Korner (DHSS 1983) and criticized the then present information systems, i.e. the type of statistics that were currently being collected concerning the community health services. The working group commented that these statistics are not as useful as they might be to managers in the context of resource allocation and planning. The proposals for reform set out in the report in many respects ignore the essential function of, for example, health visiting which involves the searching out of health needs and instead the focus is on the actual care groups visited and intervention given. However, the complexities of health visiting mean that it is difficult to categorize visits under a single heading.

Statistics concerning community health care are needed for many reasons and these have been summarized in the report as follows:

- Planning and monitoring
- Evaluation and research
- Operational control
- Treatment of individual patients/clients
- Legal requirements
- Accountability

The report concentrates on data collection to meet the needs of planning and monitoring, operational control and accountability. However, it is conceivable that the information collected may be put to other uses. The Korner report focused attention on the need for information about community nursing services, and the recommendations have been widely adopted. The issues involved in developing a community nursing information system are discussed in Chapter 6.

A further example of process evaluation is the nursing audit (Phaneuf, 1976); here, the focus is on not just what the nurse does but may also include some notion of how well she performs in her role. In the context of health visiting an audit for evaluating the performance of students or health visitors could be developed from the skills outlined in the Council for the Education and Training of Health Visitors' document 'Time to Learn' (CETHV 1982b). To use an example, if we look at the section in the report on the skills involved in interviewing we see that the 'attitudinal set' for this skill is itemized as follows:

(1) Be non-judgmental both orally and non-verbally
(2) Be willing to listen and empathize
(3) Value objectivity as appropriate (in research mode)
(4) Value subjectivity as appropriate (show human warmth)
(5) Value clients' rights to privacy and confidentiality
(6) Value goal of clients having independence

(7)   Value own listening role
(8)   Affirm the principles of the practice of health visiting.

As a nursing officer or tutor involved in the appraisal of health visitors or students we could use items 1–8 as a check list against which we could evaluate interviewing skills in either staff or students. The assumption underlying process evaluation is that what the nurse does is of primary importance and evaluations are made concerning nurse-, rather than client-orientated objectives. Furthermore this example reiterates the subjective nature of evaluation.

Outcome evaluation: outcome evaluation on the other hand refers to the end result of care in terms of its affect upon the patient or client. In brief a judgment is made about the achievement of client-orientated objectives with no regard to the reason why the observed outcome occurred. The assumption underlying outcome evaluation is that the care a person receives is of secondary importance to its effects – hence the emphasis is placed upon the patient or client and not the nurse.

Outcome evaluation is implicit in the nursing process where client-orientated goals or objectives are set and act as the criteria against which the success or failure of intervention is evaluated. In the context of community health nursing, it is usually assumed that the goals of care are commonly understood, although this is seldom the case. Where possible the expected outcome of intervention should be written down in the client or family record. The expected outcome of intervention can take many forms. It may relate to the acquisition of new knowledge as a result of a one to one teaching, or a behavioural change as in potty training or visiting the family planning clinic. Whatever the expected outcome or criteria for judging the success of the intervention it should be clearly stated so that what constitutes success or failure can be readily understood by any nurse.

Let us now consider an example: all newborn babies are at risk from developing gastroenteritis. This risk is increased if the infant is bottle-fed, if the bottle is made up for two feeds and then reheated, and if the parents have little understanding of the need for sterilization. In such circumstances the health visitor may list gastroenteritis as a potential problem.

Goal Statement A: the mother/father will demonstrate that they understand the preparation of bottle feeds and the way to sterilize bottles.

This statement has limitations because it does not indicate how the parents will demonstrate their understanding and we have no indication of the time perspective. Will it be at the next visit or for the next baby? Goal statement B gives us this additional information.

Goal Statement B: the mother/father will discuss the way in which they make up the bottle feeds and their method of sterilization and will give a practical demonstration at the next visit which has been arranged for, say, 10.00 hours on 4 April.

In the context of outcome evaluation it can be argued that in some respects community health nursing is rather more complex to evaluate than hospital nursing. In the community we are dealing with families not individuals; however, this is not intended to imply that the hospital nurses do not consider the family as important. When nurses visit clients in their own homes the focus of their work is on the family. The initial reason for the visit may have been precipitated by a referral from a general practitioner reporting the failing mental state of an elderly person. Despite the fact that the elderly person is in one sense the client, it may well be that the nurse directs most of her intervention towards the daughter who feels that she cannot go on indefinitely caring for her mother. In the context of hospital nursing a care plan is usually only made for the patient – that is, the person who occupies the bed in the ward. Hence the outcome of care is only evaluated in this context.

In community nursing it is not always so clear cut as to who the patient or client is and it may well be necessary to make more than one care plan. Similarly, goals may be in conflict with each other and many compromises will need to be made. If, for example, a woman feels she can no longer care for her mentally confused mother-in-law because she is getting little or no support from her husband then there are three individuals to consider. Any attempts to evaluate the outcome of intervention would have to take into account the conflicting needs of these three individuals. In order to begin to deal with this problem, i.e. the family's perceived inability to care for a mentally confused elderly person, the nurse might initially try to uncover the reason for the apparently sudden feelings of not being able to cope on the part of the daughter-in-law.

The community health nurse has certain beliefs and values about the function of the family and male and female roles within it. She has acquired this knowledge from her roles as a woman, as a nurse and perhaps as a health visitor or district nurse. Let us say that on taking a family history from the female carer we learn that she used to work as a cleaner and gave up work six months ago to be at home with her mother-in-law. She is in many respects happily married but considers that her husband has put pressure on her to give up work to take care of his mother. She feels that her husband is rather old-fashioned about women working and prefers her to be at home. The husband has never helped in the house but he does do all the gardening and decorating.

The situation in this household was tolerable until the husband's mother began getting up in the night and wandering around the house and out into the street. Because the husband has to be at work by 08.00 hours each morning the wife felt it was her duty to get up to keep an eye on her mother-in-law. This practice has resulted in her feeling very tired and unable to cope with the housework, shopping and cooking. The problem has been further compounded by the recent onset of urinary incontinence in the elderly person and it was when this happened that she went to her general practitioner. When speaking to the mother-in-law the health visitor finds that she is disorientated in time and place and that she repeatedly asks to be taken home to her mother. She seems not to know the name of her daughter-in-law but does remember the name of her son. Towards the end of the interview the husband returns from work and makes it quite plain that he has no intention of letting his mother go into a home or a hospital. He also considers that his wife exaggerates the problem. Clearly there is no right or obvious answer to this family's problems. Indeed, it would be interesting to identify the actual and potential problems of each family member and try to write goal statements for each. Let us say that the nurse in question considers that it is the female carer that has the most dominant or pressing needs, then what can she do to ameliorate the situation?

Decisions concerning intervention are not made in a social vacuum, they are made in the context of service cutbacks and an awareness of the constraints of time. Let us say that it is decided that a possible solution to the problem would be day care five days a week for the elderly person (something the husband is in agreement with). The problem then becomes one of getting the placement and the transport. In the first instance there may be no vacancy at all. As an interim measure the nurse has to somehow offer support to the female carer to enable her to carry on a little longer. This support may be given by providing an opportunity for her to talk about how she feels both about her marriage and caring for her mother-in-law. In addition, time may be spent with the husband to try to give him some insight into his wife's situation in the hope that he will be willing to help more in the house. The nurse may also give some practical advice and assistance with the management of the incontinence such as arranging for the laundry service and the provision of incontinence aids such as Kanga pads and pants. There may also be financial benefits that the family are entitled to such as an attendance allowance.

Obviously there are a number of other interventions that we might try but our intention here is not to provide an exhaustive list but instead to provide some insight into the complexities of dealing with families. An example of this nature introduces another problem in the context of evaluation in so far as it is not possible to evaluate what you are unable to provide, in this case, day care. Nevertheless community health nurses are in a position to collect data concerned with existing services that fall short in meeting the needs of the community. We contend that all practitioners have a moral responsibility to collate this information if they are to be serious about meeting community needs.

To return to evaluation, it is incumbant upon the evaluator to decide whether to use structure, process or outcome criteria, or a combination of two or more of these. In choosing a particular approach to evaluation certain assumptions have to be made. If it is possible in terms of time and financial resources it may be advantageous to attempt an evaluation incorporationg structure, process and outcome goals and it might be expected that there would be a positive correlation between the three approaches.

Process-outcome evaluation

An alternative approach to evaluation has been suggested by Bloch (1975), namely process-outcome evaluation. Here the study of process is related to the study of outcome.

'In process evaluation one examines and makes judgements about what is done by the care provider. In outcome evaluation one examines and makes a judgement about the achievement of patient orientated objectives. The results of the latter can be dangerously sterile, because when process is not also examined one cannot know what caused the favourable and unfavourable outcomes. Only evaluation which encompasses both process and outcome has the potential for great impact on the quality of care.' (Bloch 1975)

Nurses view the patient or client as the central figure in their work; there is therefore a great temptation to focus on outcome evaluation and some work has been done in this area (Berg, 1974; Hilger, 1974; Zimmer, 1974; Luker, 1982a). Bloch suggests that process outcome evaluation studies might be undertaken by collecting both process and outcome data for specific patient or client problems. The data may then be analysed in terms of the care given to those people who experience favourable outcomes and the care given to those people who experience unfavourable outcomes. It is thought that in this way the interventions which most frequently produce a favourable outcome might be identified and subsequently used to replace those interventions which most frequently produce an unfavourable outcome. It is suggested that such studies might be undertaken in order to obtain information and insight into how the care given to patients or clients might be improved.

An attempt at process-outcome evaluation was made by Luker (1982b) but the findings were equivocal. It became apparent that clients who shared the same problems and introduced the same variables into the situation were prescribed, at least on paper, identical interventions. This finding raised questions concerning client motivation and the influence of the micro-processes of nurse-client interaction with regard to the outcome of intervention. It would seem that the way in which community health nurses deliver their interventions in terms of style of interaction would provide a useful focus for research if related to the outcome of intervention.

Against the background of the NHS and Community Care Act (1990), a greater emphasis will be placed on outcome evaluation as evidenced by health gain. As previously stated in the introduction, District Health Authorities are charged with the responsibility of assessing the health needs of their resident population. Priorities will be set and services targeted accordingly. Performance will be measured by comparing health outcomes within and between health districts. By focusing on client, or patient outcomes, the contribution of individual practitioners in the primary health care team becomes less important since it is the collective effort which will be the measurable input in most cases. However, if community nursing services are to survive and develop it is essential that individual practitioners are in a position to identify, quantify and evaluate their own input in terms of client outcomes.

The section that follows addresses the particular issues involved in evaluating health visiting. It is necessary to single out health visiting work for special attention since it is this group of community health nurses who have traditionally had an explicit commitment to health promotion and prevention work in the community.

ADDITIONAL ISSUES IN EVALUATING THE PRACTICE OF HEALTH VISITING

When seeking to evaluate health visiting practice there is a basic problem in that the goals of health visiting are broadly stated and as such cannot easily act as criteria against which the effectiveness of practice can be measured. The health visitor's work is said to have five main aspects (CETHV 1976) which for the sake of clarity are repeated here.

(1) The prevention of mental, physical and emotional ill-health or the alleviation of its consequences
(2) Early detection of ill-health and surveillance of high-risk groups
(3) Recognition and identification of need and mobilization of appropriate resources where necessary
(4) Health teaching
(5) Provision of care; this will include support during periods of stress and guidance in cases of illness as well as the care and management of children.

The Council for the Education and Training of Health Visitors (a responsibility that is now the function of the National Boards), has issued the following statement: that 'the profession has reached a stage where, in order to develop further, it must spell out its implicit principles which ultimately predict and guide its practice' (CETHV, 1977, p. 7).

A working party was set up with the terms of reference 'to examine the principles and practice of health visiting' and a definition of health visiting was agreed upon as follows: 'the professional practice of health visiting consists of planned activities aimed at the promotion of health and the prevention of ill-health' (CETHV, 1977, p. 8).

The overall goal of health visiting can therefore be said to be 'the promotion of health and prevention of ill health'. However, this is too broad and unrealistic a goal to be considered as a single outcome criterion for health visiting practice.

Health visiting places an emphasis on prevention and therefore it shares the problems inherent in the evaluation of all preventive techniques or programmes; namely, if something does not occur because it has been prevented how can it be measured? In a discussion on measuring the effects of prevention, Lave and Lave (1977) state that the old adage 'an ounce of prevention is worth a pound of cure', is not an acceptable guide to the allocation of resources in the community because effective preventive techniques are lacking and therefore the adage is misleading since it places into one category, 'prevention', a wide variety of programmes and activities.

Some community health programmes, such as sewage disposal or screening for phenylketonuria, can be said to be highly effective or at least cost effective. Some programmes, on the other hand, such as screening for breast cancer are controversial with respect to the target population and efficacy. Programmes which depend for their success on the compliance of the client may in some circumstances not be effective. Shapiro (1977) comments on the relationship between lifestyle and health status and suggests that there is a possibility that major improvements in health status might occur through alteration in health habits such as smoking, dietary intake and exercise. The importance of lifestyle is the major thrust in the discussion paper *The Health of the Nation* (DOH 1991). Health visitors are involved in health education at both a group and an individual level. Health visitors engage in one to one health education when they visit people in their own homes or see individual clients at the clinic. Similarly if they visit schools or participate in ante-natal classes they teach groups rather than individuals and this requires a different set of skills. Very little evidence exists concerning the effectiveness of teaching undertaken by health visitors. Hobbs (1973) commented on the lack of evidence regarding the effectiveness of one to one teaching undertaken by the health visitor; almost twenty years later we are no further forward. It can be argued that the successful outcome of the health visitor's work depends to a large extent upon the co-operation or compliance of the client. The extent to which patients follow doctors' orders has been investigated, but little or no work has been carried out concerning the clients' compliance with health visiting advice. In the context of medicine the compliance studies carried out have usually focussed on the extent to which patients have followed their drug prescription. Since non-compliance has been a problem to general practitioners in so far as it has hindered the efficacy of their treatment, the quest has been to search out the potential non-complier so that he or she can be dealt with. The emphasis in these studies has been to see the problem – that is, non-compliance – from the doctor's point of view rather than the patient or client's point of view. A notable exception to this approach was the work of Stimpson (1974) whose study sought to view the issue of non-compliance from the patient's viewpoint. Stimpson (1974) concludes that rarely are medical instructions or drug prescriptions consumed in a social vacuum. Patients, in fact, evaluated doctors' orders and make decisions about whether or not to follow the advice in the light of the discussions they have with people who share their own social and cultural background. While to the best of our knowledge no work of this nature has been carried out concerning whether or not clients follow the advice given to them by health visitors, intuitively we feel that there is a high incidence of non-compliance with health visitors' advice. It would be interesting to investigate the clients' perception of health visitor advice since this may assist in improving the service to the clients.

In the days of the sanitary missionary through primary prevention it was possible to lower the infectious disease mortality and morbidity rates. Today, in the era of the generic family visitor, we are in the position of choosing among interventions which have much lower levels of effectiveness. The reason for this is that today we are dealing with more problems where the resolution can only be achieved by a fundamental change in client behaviour. The example of obesity makes this point. In order to lose weight it is necessary to alter one's eating patterns and consequently one's shopping habits. Food and the sharing of food also have social meaning and, therefore, reducing weight may require an adjustment to be made in many aspects of everyday life. Few people would be willling to alter their behaviour to this extent. The apparent lack of dramatic opportunities to measure the effects of prevention is one estimate of how far we have come in community health (Lave & Lave, 1977).

In discussing a possible model for assessing the work of the health visitor, Luker (1978) has argued as follows:

'Some health visitors believe that the effects of health visiting are too subtle, intangible or elusive to be realistically assessed. If this were so there would be little reason for health visitors to offer a service, since no one, including the client, would be aware of its effects. Intangible and elusive changes can hardly be worthwhile goals or a reason for continuing professional practice.

Moreover in the context of the present economic climate it would seem urgent to assess the care given by health visitors in order to demonstrate its effectiveness and to justify the provision of the service.'

Health visitors have been content to avoid studying the process of health visitor intervention in terms of its benefit to the client by dismissing it as methodologically impractical. Researchers have focused instead on describing health visiting in terms of what health visitors say they do (Clark, 1973; Colliety, 1988/89; Gilmore *et al.*, 1974; Henderson, 1978; Jeffreys, 1965; Marris, 1971; Poulton, 1977). In a review of literature on Primary Health Care, Hicks (1976) made the following statement:

'No one can have any excuse for not trying to evaluate the work of health visitors, although the term "support" is difficult to express in quantitative terms "ensure" is more explicit and it should be possible to test the extent to which the health visitor succeeds when she is expected to ensure this and the other.'

The preventive aspects of health visiting are difficult to measure because of the long-term nature of the work and the lack of data other than for specific programmes such as immunization and developmental screening. However, health visitors do deal with clients and families who have tangible problems which are amenable to short-term intervention. In attempting to solve short-term problems health visitors may affect the future health of the client or family in an unknown way since problems which are prevented from developing because of health visitor intervention cannot readily be assessed. Nevertheless, it is thought that evaluation of health visitor intervention in terms of its effect upon the client might begin in the area of tangible problems. Few attempts have been made to evaluate the effectiveness of health visitor intervention (Luker, 1982a); in fact little research effort in nursing generally has been directed at evaluation, possibly because of the difficulties involved in demonstrating a cause and effect relationship. Ethical issues are often raised when considering the design of a study to demonstrate a cause and effect relationship. The usual scientific approach has been to use an experimental method which may necessitate denying a control group access to the service. Health visitors have seemed reluctant to deny their service in the interest of scientific enquiry and this reluctance to evaluated practice in addition to the methodological and ethical problems raises the question 'can health visitor intervention be evaluated?'

Attempts have been made in North America to evaluate the effects of 'public health nurse' intervention. It is necessary to point out, however, that the role of the 'public health nurse' in that part of the world is a combination of both the district nurse and health visitor functions. The question of how effective public health nursing is was asked by Roberts (1962); she commented that 'the paucity of concrete evidence regarding the results of nursing services is a serious handicap to planning, evaluating and directing the total public health program as well as in the nursing aspects of that program' (Roberts, 1962). Roberts highlighted the difficulties in caring for clients with long-term illnesses where the effects of the nursing, unlike the more acute and infectious diseases, are not really reflected in reports of morbidity and mortality.

Other nurses have been interested in developing a means for community nurses to assess the effects of their care upon the client. Mayers (1972) comments that community nurses have rationalized their resistance to evaluation by explaining that the desired outcomes for each client are 'individual' factors and that it is difficult and even unwise to attempt to make generalizations. Mayers attempted to identify the criteria which nurses use to evaluate their work. She observed public health nurses at work and interviewed them informally. After each visit she asked the nurse whether she believed the client was doing well or poorly and why. The nurses most frequently seemed to use criteria related to the client's physical and mental condition – his ability to act independently and to communicate effectively. This study has contributed to knowledge about the method of studying the effectiveness of public health nurse interventions in terms of attempting to identify useful criteria against which to evaluate the outcome of intervention.

The problems of evaluating social casework are similar to the problems involved in evaluating health visiting. Social workers have been somewhat more adventurous than health visitors in using the experimental methods available. Goldberg *et al.* (1970) attempted the first controlled field experiment in Britain in the complex and diffuse area known as social casework. The target population of her study was the elderly and the study involved a comparison of the outcome of one group of clients who received the services of a trained social worker with another group who received the services of an untrained social worker. Goldberg *et al.* addressed some of the key problems in evaluation which are shared by health visitors and other nurses, namely:

(1) What constitutes success?
(2) How might success be measured?
(3) What is an improvement or deterioration and for whom is it for, the client or their family?
(4) Over what time-scale should the effects of intervention be assessed?
(5) Whose judgment should be final, the client's or the professional's?

The questions posed by Goldberg are central to any attempt at evaluation. These questions have no straightforward answers but could usefully form the basis of seminar or group work for both students and experienced health visitors. To date there is little evidence to suggest where health visitors might most usefully be deployed. It is suggested here that the opinions of experienced health visitors concerned with where they consider they have been the most and the least successful in realizing their objectives, may shed some light on the goals of health visiting practice at an individual level.

RECORD KEEPING

It may at first glance appear out of place in a chapter on evaluation to include a section on record keeping. However, it is our contention that a problem-orientated recording system may be used as an adjunct to process and outcome or process outcome evaluation.

This section is intended to assist students in presenting information in a systematic and logical way. We do not advocate that nursing records should necessarily always follow this format. Indeed, given the growing popularity of client-held records it would not be feasible for all records to follow the problem-orientated format. However, in terms of acquainting students with some of the issues involved in evaluation, we advocate this approach.

Students often comment that they have received little or no instruction on how to keep client or family records. This is often due to the fact that the tutors in colleges assume that fieldwork teachers give instruction on record keeping and yet all too often the fieldwork teachers assume that record keeping has been part of the college curriculum.

Information management is one of the core components of community health nursing. Records are important and are therefore transferred to other health districts when clients move. Records form the basis for confidential reports to other agencies and indeed act as evidence in court. In addition, they are important to managers and may be subject to audit which, as we have already mentioned, is a form of process evaluation.

Unlike hospital nursing work, community health nurses work in isolation hence their work is virtually invisible to monitoring by supervisors (Dingwall, 1977). Health visitors, for example, are seldom observed on home visitors and this provides much scope for individual variations in practice. The only area of a community health nurse's work which can readily be monitored is her record keeping. Thus, according to Dingwall, for a practitioner to demonstrate that she is performing satisfactorily she should keep adequate records which can verify that she has operated in an organizationally correct manner.

Problem-orientated recording

If community health nurses collect information from their clients in accordance with their personal philosophy of health care it does not necessarily follow that recordings other than the initial assessment will be organized in a logical way. Doctors have been using formal problem-solving for much longer than nurses; however, if we look at medical records, we invariably find that systematic recording is usually only apparent in the initial assessment, and not in the subsequent progress notes.

The concept of problem-orientated medical records was pioneered by Dr Lawrence Weed. The original intention was to use problem-orientated medical records as a means of logically organizing information around the patient's medical problem. Weed (1969) uses the patient's medical records as a tool which facilitates the accomplishment of goals for and with the patients.

In Weed's (1969) problem-orientated recording system the mnemonic SOAP stands for Subjective and Objective information about a patient problem, Assessment and Planning. To make this recording format more applicable to health visiting we suggest that subjective information should relate to what the client says about the problem. Here it is important to stress that the recording should use the client's own words rather than the health visitors' interpretation of what the client meant. The term objective should be replaced by the word observation and here the health visitor records what she observes about the problem thus observation may be objective or subjective, this of course will depend to some extent on the nature of the problem.

Since within the context of community health nursing there is no obvious format for the systematic recording of progress notes, we believe that a modified problem orientated recording system, using the SOAP system, can be used to assist the health visitor to become more objective about her work and this approach may also assist her in evaluating the outcome of intervention.

The word assessment may be confused with the initial information giving or assessment visit which is sometimes regarded as the first stage in the nursing process. Hence Luker and Orr suggest that the word analysis be used instead. This implies that the practitioner places an interpretation on her observations, in doing this she takes account of what the client has said and also what she has observed. At the initial assessment visit it is likely that the analysis section of the records will contain only a statement of the problem. It is reasonable to assume that at a first visit the community health nurse will identify an actual and potential problem on the basis of what she observes and by what the client says about a particular issue or area of concern. For the second and subsequent visits, the analysis section of the records should contain a statement indicating, on the basis of the evidence, whether or not the problem is the same, better, or worse than before. A plan is then developed of how to deal with the client's problem, or, alternatively, how to help the client deal with his or her own problem.

When writing about problem-orientated recording we are mindful of health visitors' general reluctance to consider that they are dealing with clients with problems. This approach does not ignore the preventive aspect of the work, but enhances the preventive function by requiring the nurse to make explicit her intentions in the planning section of the records. This approach also encourages community health nurses to evaluate their work, since they are obliged to write a substantial judgment of 'worth' into the analysis section of the records.

It is worth pointing out that new record cards are not necessary when the SOAP format for recording progress notes is used. It is not essential to write out the problem and goal each time an entry is made. If the problems and goals are numbered then the number will be all that is required. It may be helpful at this point to include an example of problem-orientated records using the modified SOAP format.

Example

This example concerns an elderly lady who was referred to the health visitor by the general practitioner. Her problem was identified as 'difficulty in losing weight'. It was important for this client to reduce her weight because of underlying medical pathology which it was thought would improve if the client lost 2 st in weight.

Front of record card:

Problem: difficulty in losing weight

Goals: to reach target weight of 10 st

Progress notes:

First visit – 1.2.92

S: 'I would like to lose a bit of weight, the doctor says I must. I am about 11 st 10 lb and that's too much. I don't seem to be able to take it off.'

O: Client looks overweight: dress very tight, stockings don't go much over the knee.
     Weight 12 st 2 lb.

A: Really does seem interested in losing weight.

P: (1)   Provide client with list of forbidden foods and foods high in refined carbohydrates.

     (2)   Weigh at monthly intervals and plot weight on a graph. Stick graph on kitchen cupboard door.

     (3)   Discuss meal planning and plan menu for a week with the client.

3.3.92

S: 'I am a bit heavy but I don't seem able to lose it. I am trying.'

O: Weight 12 st 2 lb: eager to discuss diet and high refined carbohydrate foods which should be avoided.

A: Has gained weight possibly because she is unsure about what foods to avoid.

P: (1)   Discuss foods which should be avoided and write down in list form.

     (2)   Same as for P 2 and P 3 of last visit.

3.4.92
S: 'I have been seeing to my son, he is not well, he is a diabetic. I have had a lot of running about lately.'
O: Weight 11 st 9 lb. Encouraged by this.
A: Lost 7 lb since last month probably due to increase in exercise and anxiety about son.
P: (1) Discuss the value of exercise in conjunction with diet.
    (2) Weigh and encourage.

4.5.92
S: 'I do try not to eat too much. I don't take sweet things. I keep on the move. I see to my son and make his dinner.'
O: Weight 11 st 7 lb, taking daily exercise, understands diet.
A: Lost total 9 lb in 4 months. Weight coming off very slowly.
P: (1) Continue monthly weighing but invite to clinic. No further home visits unless her weight goes back on.
    (2) Discuss the possibility of the client going to *Weight Watchers*.

This example gives a good insight into how the nurse was attempting to deal with this client's problem and the record also clearly states the progress the client made. Some practitioners feel that this type of record keeping is too time consuming to be used on day-to-day practice. Those of us who have used this method have found it time consuming at first but once we have become used to the approach we are surprised at how adept we become. It is suggested that community health nurses might be encouraged in the first instance to use this style of recording for selected problems such as infant feeding problems or obesity. This would mean that they would develop some competence in recording in this way and may then think it worthwhile to extend it to other aspects of their work. It is thought that as a learning exercise students should be encouraged to use problem-orientated recording in their family or care studies. This approach to record keeping can also provide useful data about how community health nurses approach particular client problems. If the analysis section of the record is filled in adequately we may also gain an insight into the outcome of the intervention. This type of information can be used retrospectively and may in some cases constitute evaluative research.

CONCLUSION

In the context of the 'purchaser provider ideology', value for money as evidenced by health gain is the currency in the market place. Health visitors and other community health nurses have thus been forced to reflect on their contribution to health care.

It is evident that in the past community health nurses have been reluctant to evaluate their work. Instead they have been content to claim that a meaningful evaluation was impossible, due to the individual nature of client problems and the centrality of the relationship with the client. Owing to competing demands on services and restricted financial resources at a national and local level there is an inherent danger in community health nurses attempting to spread themselves across all client groups. On the one hand, by taking on more work, i.e. claiming to visit more at risk groups such as the unemployed, the bereaved, the handicapped and the elderly, the service is in a prime position to compete for additional financial resources within each health district. However, the stumbling block to this expansion policy is that, when challenged, managers have little evidence readily available to substantiate the claim that benefit would be accrued by appointing more qualified practitioners in a particular area. Whilst community health nurses might believe that they do 'good work' this is no longer sufficient evidence to be convincing to others who may be sceptical about the benefit of the service. In order to secure continued or additional resources community health nurses should be prepared to generate information about what they do and the outcome of their work.

6 Information Technology and Community Health Nursing

Maria Kenrick, MSc, BSc(Hons), RGN, *Research Assistant, Research and Development Unit, Department of Nursing, University of Liverpool*

INFORMATION TECHNOLOGIES IN CONTEXT

The collection and dissemination of information is already a central aspect of community health nursing and all practitioners are likely to find that information technology (IT) will become increasingly important in their work.

IT is primarily a management tool, used to provide the facilities for functional budgeting and operational and strategic planning. Its use, however, is now becoming more widespread and in the recent past the use of IT systems in health care has become common.

It is appropriate to review the development of health service IT in the context of the legislation which has substantially altered the organizational culture and philosophy of the NHS. It is also useful to consider the professional issues raised by existing and potential IT applications in community health locations.

IT is commonly believed to be concerned with computer hardware and software, since this is its most sophisticated application. However, IT literally refers to any technological means by which information is stored, transmitted or processed. There are many existing IT applications which have been assimilated into everyday life and are already an integral part of community nursing practice.

Audio and video tapes are perhaps the most obvious in this regard, and these have a useful function in health education. Many ante-natal clinics routinely show videos of labour and delivery to pregnant women, and there are numerous audio and video recordings available which contain information on health-related issues such as dieting, exercise programmes and relaxation techniques.

Health service records have been stored for many years on microfilm, and more recently on compact discs. Although many health profession als have no need of microfilmed records, these same technologies are widely employed for maintaining catalogues in public libraries, and any library user will probably be familiar with these techniques. Some community health nurses may already be using tape recorders or electronic organizers as a means of keeping temporary records, and most professionals will at some time have recourse to a facsimile (fax) machine for the transmission of printed information.

Magnetic memory cards are another aspect of IT which is in everyday use. Many adults have bank or credit cards on which a small amount of information about the holder is stored on a magnetic strip on the back of the card. When inserted into an appropriate decoder these strips can be read and a financial transaction effected. Work is being undertaken in Britain and Europe to explore the potential of magnetic and microchip cards as means of storing patient records, and these are discussed below.

Word processing equipment is part of the standard office furniture of many organizations, and ownership of home computers is widespread. Many community health nurses will be familiar with the techniques of processing information in this way. Larger computer systems have been in use in the health service since the early 1960s and have a variety of clinical and financial applications such as EMI scanners and computerized ledgers (Barber & Scholes, 1979).

Within the community health setting, computer systems are used for such purposes as administering child immunization programmes. Master patient indexes have also been developed to monitor population movements and health status. Although nurses may not have had direct experience of existing health service computer applications, this situation is unlikely to persist much longer. The Department of Health (DOH) Information Management Group Working Party on Community Health Services (1990) reported that over 50% of GP practices had installed computer systems, and of those that had not, computerization of practice administration and records was a priority target for the following year.

Given that information technologies are an integral part of everyday life and have been in use in the NHS for a considerable time, the question raised is why the current development of health service IT should be an issue for health professionals.

IT IN THE NHS

Review of the literature suggests that IT systems include both the techniques and equipment for handling information and the people who use them (WHO, 1988). The notion of technological systems having a human element is an important one, and there is a considerable body of evidence which indicates that the introduction of IT to the workplace has both behavioural and attitudinal consequences.

Wall (1987) suggests that new technologies can fundamentally alter either the mental or physical components of a job, and are therefore potentially threatening to workers. Depending on the nature of the work being done, IT may either enhance or limit working behaviours. For example, a study by Buchanan and Boddy (1983) found that technological innovations in a particular manufacturing organization had the effect of deskilling one group of employees while enlarging the jobs of another group. At the organizational level the introduction of new technology is invariably associated with some reorganization of occupational roles and working relationships. Access to information is believed to be one of the mechanisms for exerting power in an organization (Handy, 1988) and it is possible to visualize the situation in a health centre where only the records clerk knows how to use the computer – and the effects this could have on working roles and relationships.

The pace of change and the underlying purpose of IT developments in the NHS also have implications for community health nurses. Fox (1987) suggests that the speed at which new technologies are assimilated has a crucial bearing on the outcome of implementation. Theoretically, domestic applications of IT are within the control of the individual who alone dictates the pace of change. As anyone who has purchased a home computer or video recorder will know, once the processes of choosing, rationalizing and learning are completed, these applications are rarely threatening or incomprehensible.

A major difference between domestic IT applications and the implementation of IT in the Health Service is in the nature of the latter being part of a massive organizational change which is largely beyond the experience of control of individual nurses (Zielstorff, 1984; Bowman, 1986). Perhaps more significantly, the Health Service IT developments are the tangible elements of a shift in the organizational philosophy toward a financially driven and management-oriented service, something which could have profound consequences for all professional practices.

NHS REORGANIZATION

As a member of the World Health Organisation, the UK is committed to the goal of 'Health for All by the Year 2000', with its emphasis on the provision of primary health care (WHO 1978). Changes in the structure of the NHS are being determined by the NHS and Community Care Act (1990), which embraces the concept of an internal market for care provision, with financial viability becoming a key objective for all professional staff. A central feature of the legislation is that the distribution of health resources be based on factual data rather than perceived need (Millar, 1989), and to this end the Act envisages the widespread implementation of IT systems in all health care locations.

The 1990 NHS Act makes a distinction between health and social care without delineating responsibility for provision and funding of these services. Although the role of the NHS remains essentially unaltered, Health Authorities and Family Health Service Authorities (FHSAs), will be expected to make specific contributions to the arrangements for community care, previously the responsibility of Local Authorities (Miller & Sheldon, 1989). The Act also identifies the need for a 'key worker' who will be responsible for the assessment and co-ordination of an individual's health and social needs.

Given the professional backgrounds of Health Visitors and District Nurses, their association with general medical practices and their links with social service agencies (Orr, 1985), it would be logical to suppose that they are well qualified to assume this 'key worker' role. However, experienced nurses are an expensive health commodity, and with the economic philosophy underpinning this legislation they will be increasingly required to justify their practices and to demonstrate the financial viability of the services they provide. This requirement could present a serious threat to the continuation of the community health nurse's role. As Luker (1985) argues, the nature of nursing work in the community makes systematic evaluation of practice both necessary and problematic.

As part of the NHS reforms, a new contract for General Practitioners was introduced in April 1990. Consistent with the concepts of 'health for all' and the increasing financial emphasis on health care, GPs are remunerated for their work in health education and disease prevention and for monitoring the health and social welfare of the elderly. They are also expected to provide immunization programmes and child health and development services, and to offer health screening to 'at risk' groups in the population. All these services are commonly thought to be the work of health visitors and district nurses. However, with the devolution of responsibility and finances down to FHSA and group practice level, it is debatable whether the continued provision of community nursing services in their current form could be made.

The introduction of contracts for the purchase and provision of health services will have an effect on the working practices of all health professionals, and it seems that some change in the roles of health visitors and community nurses is inevitable. The two extreme possibilities are that within the new style NHS the function of the community health nurse will be completely eroded; alternatively, it could become central to the primary health care team (Fatchett, 1990).

The increasing use of IT systems for contract administration is likely to present community health nurses with some practical and theoretical difficulties. Most existing Health Authority information systems are concerned with collecting task-related or 'activity analysis' data. The inherent reductionism of these systems renders them unable to account for the complexity of a particular intervention, and hence it is very difficult to evaluate the 'efficiency' of nursing practices.

Computerized information systems will also open community health nursing to scrutiny by people outside the profession. While this in itself is not necessarily a problem, general managers and accountants will be concerned that providing nursing care is an efficient and cost effective way of meeting service targets. In this case it is important that information collected about nursing activity accurately reflects the processes and outcomes of nursing practice.

It is apparent that the effects of IT implementation in the Health Service are complex. Barnard *et al.* (1981) suggest that the majority of new IT users need not be concerned with developing computer skills, but should consider technological systems as a resource to be used in pursuit of the wider objectives of their profession. The alternative to this is that groups of health professionals who do not accommodate the new technologies may find themselves marginalized and their practice determined by the assumptions of 'computer experts'.

Theoretically, the development of IT in the community will provide nurses with an invaluable tool with which to monitor, develop and evaluate their practice. However, the available evidence suggests that the successful use of IT systems is dependent on a number of organizational and attitudinal factors and that the effects of IT implementation are not easily predictable. Given the nature of community nursing work it would be difficult to determine whether IT developments will ultimately enhance or limit practice.

THE DEVELOPMENT OF NHS INFORMATION STRUCTURES

The necessity for health service information systems and their associated technical applications can be understood when considered in the context of the global strategy for health care (WHO 1978), the continuing search for better management of the NHS, and the ongoing development of the silicon chip.

The report of the WHO Primary Health Care Information Technology

Working Group (1988) demonstrated that the adequacy of available management information was a problem for all member states. Despite there being an abundance of health data, its usefulness was generally inhibited by low reliability, untimeliness and inappropriate interpretation. The working group suggested that information systems were essential for the effective delivery of health services, and that collection of data should be carried out at the point of service delivery.

The Korner reports

The limitations of the NHS information networks have been long recognized and successive government reviews of the structure of the Health Service have criticized the adequacy of existing information systems (DHSS 1972; DHSS 1979). In 1980 the Steering Group on Health Services Information was established under the chairmanship of Edith Korner. The remit of the group was to examine the whole field of health statistics, and recommend a strategy for data collection and interpretation which would allow for improvement in the management of the service in terms of resource allocation and outcome measures. Prior to this, data collection was determined by Department of Health requirements, and the Korner reports were important in their acknowledgement of the need for information to be relevant to local service providers.

The Korner committees examined information needs in relation to hospital clinical activity (1982), patient transport services (1984), manpower (1984), activity in hospitals and the community (1984), services for and in the community (1985), and health services finance (1985).

The approach of the Korner groups was to identify the amount and type of data that would be required by a District Health Authority to plan, deliver and evaluate its services. The assumption was that this amount of information would also be relevant to Regional Health Authorities, the Department of Health, and local service managers, and would therefore facilitate resource allocation and valid comparisons between districts. Perhaps more significantly, the Korner reports identified the need for 'minimum data sets' (mds) specific to different types of activity in the NHS. They defined the minimum data set (DHSS 1985, p. 5) as

'. . . the data without which an HA and its management team would be handicapped in the discharge of their duty to plan, monitor and account for the services for which they are responsible.'

The committee recommended that the minimum data sets be capable of routine collection as a by-product of operational procedures, and should not therefore generate extra work for those delivering community health services. Another important element of the Korner reports was their vision of a computerized, networked information system in the NHS which would allow live interrogation of the database and would generate immediate and relevant information. To this end, the minimum data sets were made appropriate to both manual and computerized information systems.

The fifth Korner report (1985) sought to present a view of community health information systems which would integrate with hospital, para-medical and social services. The committee also made an important distinction between services *for* the community, and patient care *in* the community, the former being largely the remit of health visitors and the latter the work of district nurses.

While recognizing the complexity of nursing work in the community, the report moved away from the concept of collecting staff activity information and recommended that information about services for and in the community be related to individual client contacts. They also proposed that community health services information be organized into four broad programme types: immunization, health surveillance and early detection of disease; health promotion and education; professional advice and support; and patient care programmes. So, for example, a developmental assessment of a pre-school child would be classified as part of a health surveillance programme while post-natal care of a mother would constitute professional advice and support. Korner also recommended that each of the four programme types should have an annual statement of objectives, a defined target population, an estimate of expenditure, and a record of contacts made. The purpose of categorizing nursing work in this way was not to delimit practice, but rather to use this information, together with that from the Office of Population Censuses and Surveys (OPCS), local government agencies and hospitals, to ascertain whether health targets were being met and appropriate populations being reached.

The Korner reports generally had a mixed reception; however, all health authorities were instructed to implement the recommendations by April 1987.

The main concern for practitioners was the fact that reducing information about community health nursing to a series of programmes did not account for the complexity of practice. Although this may be a valid criticism, the purpose of the report was to standardize management information and not to devise a framework for a professional information system. It is arguable that management information needs are quite different from, and may even run counter to, professional aspirations.

The Joint Working Group of the Korner Committee and the Faculty of Community Medicine (Knox, 1987), while welcoming the main recommendations of the fifth report, also expressed concern about the oversimplification of community health services information. They suggested that standardized management information and inter-district comparisons took no account of regional variations in health status and needs. The Joint Working Group anticipated that improved management information would shift responsibility for the allocation of health resources and undermine the primacy of the medical profession.

Despite professional concerns about the consequences of implementation, the Korner reports have undoubtedly had two important effects. Firstly, the recommendations represent a serious attempt to rationalize health information needs and to improve validity and relevance of information. The Korner minimum data sets are also used as the basis of the patient specific data sets described by the NHS Information Management Group in their 'Framework for Information Systems' proposals (1990).

Secondly, the Korner reports have stimulated research within the nursing profession directed toward defining and measuring the constituents of nursing work. For example, as a direct result of implementing the Korner recommendations, a London HA attempted to quantify and cost health visiting and district nursing practice. The community management unit conducted a three-day survey of a 20% sample of the health visiting population and a 21% sample of district nursing staff. Data were collected on number and types of contacts, age groups of clients, types of skills deployed and work generated by contacts, number of failed contacts, client dependency levels, group activities and clerical work undertaken (Speakman, 1984). Unfortunately, the survey only produced a frequency analysis and a broad description of how these groups of staff had spent their working day. However, surveys such as these raise questions which have relevance to all nurses. Given the nature of community health work, how much and what type of information is necessary to cost and manage a community nursing service; do concepts such as patient dependency serve any useful purpose in attempts to quantify practice? It may be the case that attempts to measure nursing work only serve to illustrate a fundamental difference in the values and objectives of professionals and managers.

The reports of the Korner committees coincided with the publication of the findings of the NHS Management Inquiry (DHSS 1983). Although the Griffiths Report was primarily concerned with proposals for new management arrangements in the health service, it also acknowledged the need for information systems and technologies which would facilitate the strategic and operational management of the service.

Griffiths envisaged a health service which was managed rather than administered, and as a result the NHS has undergone a radical rearrangement of the organizational culture to a management-oriented service where concepts such as 'quality assurance', 'productivity' and 'performance indicators' are an integral part of health care provision.

The Korner and Griffiths reports had major implications for the definition and organization of NHS information structures, not only because of their content, but also because of their timing. The rationalization of health information needs and management arrangements in the early 1980s coincided with enormous technical advances in the IT field which made these applications accessible to even the smallest organizations. It is conceivable that this wider cultural development added momentum to the changes being introduced into the NHS.

The resource management initiative

A direct consequence of the Korner and Griffiths reports was the introduction of management budgeting experiments. Service units were encouraged to develop budgets, together with clinicians, which related workload and service objectives to financial and manpower targets (DHSS 1983). The central element of these experiments was the provision and utilization of accurate information.

In 1986, Management Budgeting evolved into the Resource Management Initiative (RMI), the stated purpose of which (DHSS 1986) was as follows:

'To enable the NHS to give a better service to patients by helping clinicians and other managers to make better informed judgements about how the resources they control can be used to maximum effect.'

Theoretically, the RMI has brought together the concepts of cost effectiveness, management processes and information provision, and established them as necessary elements of health service provision (Buxton, Packwood & Keen, 1989).

Resource Management (RM) projects were piloted in six acute hospitals and two community health units. Pilot sites established different management structures and were responsible for determining local information needs. The DHSS (1986) reported that although the two community units had adopted very different management structures and information systems, the collection of data at the level of individual patient contacts had substantially improved the operational management of both these community health service units. They also reported that the development of information networks had resulted in clearer demarcation of responsibility and accountability between general practitioners, health visitors, district nurses and paramedical staff. As part of the second phase of the initiative, RM programmes have been implemented in several community units in ten health regions.

The RMI programme has not proved entirely successful, despite the fact that the Government has been ideologically committed to this project and has invested large amounts of money in the pilot sites. As information systems and technologies are fundamental to the success of the RMI, much of the extra funding has been spent on IT applications which are increasingly found to be inappropriate for the users' information needs.

As an example of this, the investigation by Buxton *et al.* (1989) of IT applications in the RM pilot sites found that many commercially developed systems were data rich and information poor and had very limited practical application. Research by Coombs and Cooper (1989) identified the problems associated with IT applications in the health service to be technical, financial and political. They suggest that the cost of installation of appropriate information technologies are consistently underestimated, and whereas health service managers may view information systems as essential management tools, clinicians have little belief in the ability of IT to enhance patient care. Politically, IT applications open the debate about whose information needs the systems are serving and – ultimately – who is controlling the provision of health services.

'Working for patients'

In spite of substantial reservations about the adequacy and appropriateness of available information systems, the government white papers 'Working for Patients' (1989a) and 'Promoting Better Health' (1989b) set an ambitious timetable for reform of the NHS. The dominant theme of these working papers is the requirement for efficient and effective information systems.

Besides the need to develop appropriate community health information systems, perhaps two of the more significant changes arising out of the 1990 NHS Act are the allocation of financial resources to FHSAs and GP budget holders, and the establishment of an internal market for care provision, with the delineation of purchasers and providers of health services. Both purchasers and providers need contractual specifications of the range, type, quality and cost of services to be provided, together with a mechanism for ensuring that specifications are met and invoices paid. Freeman (1990) reports that as information systems will have a central role in the post review NHS, the Information Management Group (IMG) of the NHS Executive Board have devised a framework for information systems which attempts to relate IT developments to the 'corporate objectives' of the health service.

The IMG Working Party on Community Health Services (1990) recommend that in order to meet contracting arrangements, all FHSAs and probably all GP practices will need to install computer-based systems. They also suggest that the Korner minimum data sets, with the addition of a unique patient identifier (such as their NHS number), a GP code and a contract identification code would meet the information needs of the internal market.

The IMG report (1990) recommends that all community health information becomes patient based and is collected at the point of service delivery. This recommendation will undoubtedly have implications for all community health nurses, whether they are collecting data manually or learning to use new technologies. The orientation of existing systems towards providing management information suggests that if nurses want to see health IT systems that incorporate a professional dimension then they will have to be responsible for defining their own working practices and information needs.

IT APPLICATIONS IN COMMUNITY HEALTH SERVICES

The reform of the NHS and the creation of an internal market for care provision has stimulated a growing need for networked information systems. In order to remain 'competitive', providers of health care will need to supply daily information on prices and availability of services, and purchasers wishing to secure a 'good deal' for their patients will need some means of accessing providers' information. This has inevitably opened up a very lucrative market for computer manufacturers and software designers (Coombs & Cooper, 1989).

Although community-based information systems such as 'FIP' and 'Comcare' have been in use for some years, in future, the health service is likely to be flooded with information systems and their associated technologies. The ability to evaluate such systems, in terms of their relevance to the organization and to the delivery of community nursing services, will probably become a skill demanded of all practitioners.

As a direct result of the introduction of the NHS internal market, the central elements of information systems are likely to be their accounting functions, and the question of 'costing' nursing practice will undoubtedly become a major professional issue.

FIP and Comcare

The Financial Information Project (FIP 1980) aimed to assess the feasibility of individual patient costings as the basis of management information. The original field trial of FIP in community health services developed computerized patient-based record systems for four distinct health programmes: district nursing, health visiting services to the elderly population, nursing equipment loans, and district incontinence services. All information was collected by practitioners and data from nurses' diary sheets, health assessment schedules and equipment requests formed the inputs to a central computer. Classifications of different nursing activities were consistent with the Korner categorizations. Despite the fact that the FIP trials required a total reorganization of nursing documentation, it is claimed that the use of the system significantly improved the operational management of community health services (Saddington, 1984). Since the original trials, several community health software programmes have been developed and distributed by the project, and many community nurses will be familiar with the FIP system.

Comcare is another community health information system which is widely used. The main purpose of Comcare is to facilitate service planning and utilization of health resources (Creasy, 1987). This system also relies on district nurses and health visitors collecting information for inputing to a central computer. Clarke (1986) claims that Comcare is an invaluable management tool which allows for efficient and effective staff deployment.

Both FIP and Comcare are essentially management information systems, and although patient-based costings may be essential information for the functioning of the internal market, it is the assumptions underlying the 'costings' of community nursing services which should be scrutinized. Likewise, the belief that computer-generated information is objective needs to be challenged. For example, both FIP and Comcare rely on a professional assessment of patient dependency as an indication of nursing workload.

Clarke (1986) suggests that comparing client dependancy at the time of first contact against their dependancy at the time of discharge provides not only a measure of nursing costs, but also an indication of health outcomes.

This proposition has two serious flaws: one that patient dependancy is a useful analogue of nursing work, and the other that attaining health targets implies a reduction in client dependancy.

Although the concept of dependancy may have a persuasive appeal to many nurses, as a workload index it has been criticized on philosophical, methodological and technical grounds (Gault, 1982; Barr & Moores, 1982; Miller, 1985; DHSS 1986). For example, Dylak (1991) suggests that complicated statistical formulae, based on dependancy estimations, have only a spurious relationship to actual workload, and as a planning tool they are generally unreliable. He also proposes that the assumptions about nursing which support the concept of dependancy bear little relation to the reality of practice.

The supposed relationship between patient dependancy and nursing workload has yet to be conclusively demonstrated and yet these methods are commonly used as the workload measure in both management and nursing information systems. As information systems become more widespread in community health services the issue of workload measurement will become crucial as it will directly influence the way nursing resources are deployed. The problem for the profession would appear to be one of defining the elements of practice and reconciling professional objectives to the 'corporate goals' of a financially driven health service.

An alternative approach – the teamwork system

Some attempt to address this issue has been made by a research project in the north western RHA (Bagust, Prescott & Smith, 1988). Although the study was initially hospital-based it has now been extended to cover the work of all community health nurses (Cowie, 1991).

The study was initiated in 1987, its original purpose was to compare and evaluate the commonly used dependancy-based staffing methodologies, 'Criteria for Care' and the 'Brighton Method', with a view to recommending the implementation of one approach throughout the region. The two techniques were applied on twenty medical and surgical wards in five health districts, and although both were found to have serious flaws, the data collected were scrutinized and used to generate a radically different staffing methodology. By analysis of *actual* staffing levels on wards when nurses had justed the care to be 'good', it was found that a relationship between simple objective workload measures and nurse hours existed. This can be represented by the folowing equation:

Nurse hours required = Ward overhead
                       + a × number of patients
                       + b × number of patient movements
                       + c × number of theatre cases

(*Note:* the ward overhead and the coefficients a, b and c are fixed numbers derived from the data using regression analysis.)

The underlying assumptions of the system are contrary to the philosophy underpinning dependancy studies. Teamwork is based on the premise that it is wards rather than individual patients which are staffed and that irrespective of the number of patients a certain amount of nurse time is required to manage a clinical area. The system also recognizes that nursing is a complex process and that nursing interventions often occur simultaneously with other interventions to the same patient and to other patients on the ward.

Perhaps the most important element of this approach is the credence given to professional judgment. The system assumes that nurses are able to evaluate all the factors contributing to the workload on any given span of duty and thus determine how these have affected the overall quality of nursing care delivered. Within this model of workload estimation, professional judgment is the fulcrum on which patient activity and staff hours data are balanced.

When the above research was extended to community health locations the assumption – that community nurses could evaluate overall service quality on any given shift – held. The study also proposed that a certain amount of time would be necessary to manage a caseload, irrespective of number of clients, and that a single patient contact may generate several types of nursing work. It was also suggested that contact type and location would be important factors in determining community nursing workload and would be demonstrated in the professional judgment of the quality of service delivered. This method, which was developed by a health visitor, may be used for patient-based costings but differs from other systems in that the costs and quality of community nursing services are based on professional judgments rather than managerial or technological assumptions. Like most information systems this method also has its limitations but it is important in that it moves away from patient dependancy as the central theoretical proposition and appears to provide information which is credible to both nurses and managers.

OTHER ELEMENTS OF NURSING INFORMATION SYSTEMS

Professionally, the workload assessment element is of central importance in health information systems and in the majority of 'off the shelf' nursing systems computerized care planning and staff rostering functions are linked to the workload assessment measure. Hoy (1990) suggests that the main strength of these facilities is in their ability to produce documentation quickly and easily. However, many commercially available care planning packages require a substantial input from the users before they can be operated, and if existing recording procedures are inadequate then a computerized system of itself will not improve them. Although the utility of computerized care planning, rostering and workload assessment is debatable, computer technologies obviously have considerable potential in the record keeping, information exchange and health education functions of community health nurses.

THE ELECTRONIC CARD TECHNOLOGIES

The NHS Information Management Group (1990) advocate the use of electronic card technologies in community health locations. Electronic cards, which are similar to credit cards, have either a magnetic strip or a microchip for storing patient information. Both of these are activated through a microcomputer. Magnetic strip cards have a limited memory capacity and are only capable of storing basic patient details; however, they may have some use as health identification cards.

The so-called 'smart cards', which contain a microchip, are capable of retaining approximately 11 pages of information which can be accessed by hand-held or desktop computers (Wise, 1991). These obviously have a potential use in the maintenance of health records. A computerized information system for community health services is described by Wiseman (1990) who proposes that the principle of the system is the development of a continuous, transportable care record. Theoretically, this record would be retained by the patient and all contacts or treatments would be recorded by community health staff equipped with portable microcomputers. At the end of a working day, stored information could be printed as a hard copy and also downloaded onto a central computer located at the nurse's base. Despite the cost of implementing such technology an electronic card system has considerable potential for improving record keeping and information management. It is also possible that a centralized database could provide a facility for auditing of community health nursing practices and outcomes.

COMPUTER-ASSISTED LEARNING

Another area where information technologies may impact on a community health nurse's work is in computer-assisted learning (CAL), both for staff training and development purposes and for health education.

Morrison and Betts (1990) report on a CAL project in Wessex RHA which was designed to develop nursing staff's computer awareness and skills. They describe two learning levels, both of which explore uses of wordprocessing packages, spreadsheets and simple databases. The researchers report a large increase in computer literacy amongst staff and indicate that the project has developed a function in general nurse education, with tutors using computers for instructional purposes and as audio visual supports. It is reasonable to suppose that even if the issues of workload measurement and costing are not resolved, the computerization of administrative functions and communication pathways in community health services are inevitable. In this case the development of computer awareness and skills will be a specific learning need for many community nurses, and CAL programmes such as these may prove increasingly useful.

CAL also has potential for use in health education programmes. Luker and Caress (1989) investigated the application of a CAL programme in a hospital renal unit, and suggest that although the technique of CAL in patient education is in its infancy, it appears that it can encourage patient learning through self-directed study supported by teaching from nursing staff.

It would appear that the introduction of information technologies into community health services has considerable potential for enhancing practitioners' information management and communication skills. However, in order to exploit this potential, nurses will need to analyse the adequacy of existing sources of information and determine how additional information may be used and what effect, if any, it will have on the management of a caseload.

THE INTERACTION OF ATTITUDES AND TECHNOLOGY

There is a considerable amount of literature which indicates that the attitudes of potential users of IT systems are crucial in determining the success of such applications. Much of the research has been carried out in relation to the attitudes of hospital nurses, and the small amount examining community applications has tended to focus on GPs and practice administrators (Whitehouse, 1981). However, the findings indicate some issues which may also be relevant to community nurses.

Some early work by Friel, Reznikoff and Rosenberg (1969) suggested that nurses' attitudes to IT were a function of their age and education. Their results also demonstrated significant differences between men's and women's attitudes, with female nurses being the least favourably disposed to computer applications. A study by Startsman and Robinson (1972) compared the computer-related attitudes of a large cross-section of hospital employees in different staff groups. Seven subject groups were compared across three factors representing a general evaluation of computers, willingness to use IT, and the perceived threat to job security posed by computer systems. The findings indicated that although nurses could appreciate the potential value of computers, they were the least willing to use new technologies and felt the most threatened by their implementation. The significance of human factors in health care information system applications was studied by Thies (1975). His results suggested that women employees, nurses, and personnel with no previous computer experience were significantly more likely to have negative attitudes toward computerization than other occupational groups. He also found a significant deterioration in computer-related attitudes after implementation of systems.

Although these various findings may seem ominous, Thies (1975) also proposed that computer related attitudes may be constructively modified. More recent research indicates that this is in fact the case. For example, Krampf and Robinson (1984) found no significant differences in computer-related attitudes attributable to age, education or previous computer experience and suggested that nurses' attitudes toward IT were generally positive. Sultana (1990) also found that these variables did not have any influence on nurses' attitudes, but her results showed that subjects' attitudes were essentially negative. Nurses in Sultana's study generally held the view that computer applications in clinical practice did not increase efficiency or improve patient care.

Several researchers have developed instruments to measure nurses' computer-related attitudes, but these studies have also been located primarily in hospital environments. The specifications on Stronge and Brodt's (1985) attitude measure include job security, quality of patient care, willingness to use technology, capabilities of computer systems and perceived benefits to the institution. Schwirian *et al.* (1989) modified Stronge and Brodt's scale to investigate computer-related attitudes of trained nurses and nursing students. The factors they examined were changes over time, prior experience with computers, and general attitudes toward technology. Their results indicate that nurses' attitudes were generally positive and could be influenced by training and experience. Schwirian *et al.* (1989), p. 168 state the following:

'The attitudes of nurses who use automated information systems are as important as the technology itself. Nurses must be in a position, both cognitively and affectively to fully use computers in order for computer supported information management to be used effectively. However, if nurses do not believe that the computer system will help them, then they will not use it.

Computerised management of nursing information has significant potential for improving the quality and effectiveness of nursing care in all practice locations'.

The work of Thomas (1985; 1988) also indicates that the promotion of positive attitudes toward computers is essential if nursing is to benefit from developments in health care IT. It is apparent that users' attitudes are an important element of information systems. As Baron (1986) suggests, attitudes may directly affect work-related behaviours which in turn influence the functioning and outcomes of the organization. Employees who are resistant to new technologies can react by ignoring them with the result that the technology cannot function.

In community health services, the attitudes of nurses toward information technologies will be crucial, particularly as they will be the people responsible for most of the data collection upon which these systems depend.

THE DATA PROTECTION ACT

The increasing use of computers for collecting, storing, processing and distributing personal data raises issues of confidentiality and individual's rights. The 1984 Data Protection Act offers certain safeguards to people about whom information is stored on a computer. If community health nurses' records are to be computerized, they will need to be conversant with this Act.

The Data Protection Act gives individuals a right of access to computerized records and also provides a framework through which they may challenge information held about themselves, and in some cases may claim compensation. The Act only applies to automatically processed personal data, and not manual records or files. So, for example, community health nurses using electronic card technologies would have to apply for admission to the data protection register, and would also have to allow clients access to their health records if required.

Personal data is defined by the legislation as 'information recorded on a computer about a living, identifiable individual' (Data Protection Act Guideline 1; 1989). Statements of fact and expressions of opinion are personal data, but indications of the users' intentions toward the subject are not. So in terms of community nursing records, an assessment of a client as being 'overweight due to poor dietary habits and lack of understanding of nutritional principles' would constitute personal data whereas the proposed plan of nursing intervention would not.

The Data Protection Act also places obligations on data users to register their purpose in holding personal data and requires that they comply with the data protection principles. The principles state that all personal data shall:

- 'Be obtained and processed fairly and lawfully.
- Be held only for the lawful purposes described in the users' register entry.
- Be used only for those purposes and only be disclosed to those people described in the users' register entry.
- Be adequate, relevant and not excessive in relation to the purpose for which they are held.
- Be accurate and where necessary be kept up to date.
- Be held no longer than is necessary for the registered purpose.'

In addition, the Data Protection Act requires the following (Data Protection Act Guideline 4; 1989):

- 'The user is required to keep all personal data secure from disclosure, alteration or destruction.
- The data subject may gain access to their personal data and have it corrected where appropriate.'

The existence of this Act adds another dimension to the implementation of information technologies in community health services. Patients and clients who feel their rights are being abused have recourse to the Registrar, who then can enforce compliance with the data protection principles. These principles are explicit and comprehensive and can be upheld by the maintenance of good working practices and respect for patients. In this case the Data Protection Act should not present a problem to community health nurses.

CONCLUSION

It should be apparent from the preceding discussion that the introduction of information systems into the health service has implications which extend far beyond the technologies themselves.

It is fairly easy to see how IT could facilitate the management of a caseload by improving record keeping and communication networks. However, computerization does not necessarily imply that practice will be improved. There is no evidence to support the assumption that the computerization of administrative tasks will allow nurses more time to dedicate to their patients. In seeking to improve practice through the use of new technologies community health nurses will need to develop a critical awareness of the underlying purpose of information systems and should also determine that they are making optimum use of existing technologies.

Consideration of IT systems in community health locations suggests that the functional parameters of the various technologies are both a response and a stimulus to the change in the organizational culture and philosophy of the NHS. One consequence of a market-oriented health service could be that health care becomes a by-product of technology. Professional groups will be increasingly required to justify expenditure on the services they provide and computer applications will allow the work and practices of nurses to be scrutinized by other disciplines. The predominantly financial and management orientation of NHS information systems represents the values and objectives both of the Government and service managers - it has to be added that these are not necessarily the same as those of the nursing profession.

Information technologies have many potential uses in community health services, but before incorporating them into professional practice, nurses should consider how IT may enhance their work, and, indeed, whether the underlying purpose of such systems are consistent with the goals of community health nursing.

APPENDICES

Appendix 1

CASELOAD PROFILE

NAME ....

GP ATTACHMENT .... BASE ....

GP POPULATION .... CLINICS ....

GEOGRAPHICAL AREA .... SCHOOLS ....

HV ....

0-5 AGE GROUP	Social Class I	Social Class II	Social Class III	Social Class IV	Social Class V	Other
Number of Infant Health (a) 0-11 months Cards Held						
(b) 1-5 years						

BREAKDOWN OF CHILD POPULATION

1 CHILDREN IN STABLE/FUNCTIONING FAMILIES

2 CHILDREN IN PROBLEM FAMILIES

3 CHILDREN IN ONE-PARENT FAMILIES

  (a) Single Mother

  (b) Widowed Mother

  (c) Separated Mother

  (d) Divorced Mother

(e) Single Father

4 CHILDREN ON SPECIAL DEFECT REGISTER

5 CHILDREN ON SPECIAL CARE REGISTER

6 EMOTIONALLY DISTURBED CHILDREN

7 CHILDREN 'AT RISK' FOR CHILD ABUSE

   (a) Potential

   (b) Confirmed

6 + AGE GROUP

CHILDREN ON SPECIAL DEFECT REGISTER

CHILDREN ON SPECIAL CARE REGISTER

ADULTS ON SPECIAL CARE REGISTER

ADULTS PHYSICALLY HANDICAPPED

ANTE-NATAL WOMEN

ELDERLY 65–70, 71–75, 76–80, 81–85 86

CHRONIC SICK : CA., CHEST etc.

DIABETICS

TB PATIENTS

MENTALLY ILL

Appendix 2

CASELOAD PROFILE

PRACTICE LIST SIZE ....

TOTAL FIGURES 0-5   SOCIAL CLASS

I	II	III	IV	V

Families with multifactorial problems ....

One-parent families   ....

Husband away from home temporarily   ....

Children at risk from child abuse   ....

Confirmed cases of child abuse   ....

Physically handicapped child   ....

Physically handicapped parent   ....

Mentally handicapped child   ....

Mentally handicapped parent   ....

Emotionally disturbed child   ....

OTHER CATEGORIES

Elderly   ....

TB   ....

Diabetic   ....

Handicapped   ....

Mentally ill   ....

Coronary aftercare   ....

Chronically ill   ....

Other   ....

Appendix 3: Some Useful Indicators from the Census

The following are some examples of useful indicators contained in the Census.

1   Children under five
2   School-age children
3   Pensioners (males over 65, females over 60)
4   Other age characteristics (such as those over 75)
5   Marital status
6   Average household size
7   One and two person pensioner households
8   Overcrowded households (more than 1.5 persons per room)
9   Large households (5 or more persons)
10 One-parent families
11 Owner occupiers
12 Households renting from the local authority
13 Households renting privately furnished/unfurnished
14 Households lacking or sharing bath, hot water, inside WC
15 Households with exclusive use of all three amenities
16 Households not in self-contained accommodation
17 Number of unemployed – males and females by age
18 Social class derivable from socio-economic group
19 Industry in an area
20 Hours of work of all women, married women and women with children under five
21 Non-car-owning households
22 Birthplace of residents
23 Migration into and within the area

Appendix 4: Selected Official Sources of Statistical Information

Central Office of Information
  Annual Report
Central Statistical Office
  Abstract of Regional Statistics (England, Wales, Scotland, N. Ireland)
  Annual Abstract of Statistics
  Facts in Focus
  Financial Statistics
  The General Household Survey
  List of Principal Statistical Series and Publications
  Monthly Digest of Statistics
  National Income and Expenditure
  Social Trends
  Statistical News
  UK Balance of Payments
Department of Education and Science
  Statistics of Education
Department of Employment
  Gazette
Department of Energy
  Digest of UK Energy Statistics
Department of Finance (N. Ireland)
  Digest of Statistics
  Social and Economic Trends in N. Ireland
Department of Health
  Annual Report
  Children in Care in England and Wales
  Digest of Health and Personal Social Services Statistics
  Health and Personal Social Services Statistics
  Hospital Costing Returns
  On the State of Public Health
  Report on Health and Social Subjects
  Report on Public Health and Medical Subjects
  Statistical and Research Report Series

Department of the Environment
  Digest of Environmental Pollution Statistics
  Housing and Population
  Rates and Rateable Values in England and Wales
General Register Office, Scotland
  Annual Estimates of the Population of Scotland
  Annual Report
  Weekly returns
Office of Population Censuses and Surveys (OPCS)
  Abortion Statistics
  Annual Reports
  Birth Statistics
  Cancer Statistics
  Census 1981
  Electoral Statistics
  Hospital In-Patient Enquiry
  International Migration
  Local Authority Vital Statistics
  Marriage and Divorce Statistics
  Mortality Statistics
  Population Estimates
  Population Projections
  Registrar General's Annual Estimates of Population
  Registrar General's Decennial Supplements
  Registrar General's Quarterly Returns
  Registrar General's Statistical Review
  Registrar General's Weekly Returns
  Statistics of Infections Diseases
Organisation for European Cooperation and Development (OECD)
  Economic Outlook
  Economic Surveys
  Financial Statistics
  Foreign Trade Statistics
World Health Organisation (WHO)
  World Health Statistics Annual
  World Health Statistics Report

Appendix 5: Recommendations from the Report of the Community Nursing Review (Cumberlege Report 1986), London, HMSO

1 Each district health authority should identify within its boundaries neighbourhoods for the purposes of planning, organising and providing nursing and related primary care services.
2 A neighbourhood nursing service (NNS) should be established in each neighbourhood
3 Each neighbourhood nursing service should be headed by a manager chosen for her management skills and leadership qualities, and she should be based in the neighbourhood.
4 Community midwives, community psychiatric nurses and community mental handicap nurses should ensure, through their respective managers and the neighbourhood nursing manager, that their specialist contributions are fully co-ordinated with the work of the neighbourhood nursing service.
5 All other specialist nurses who work outside hospital should be based in the community and managed as part of the neighbourhood nursing service. Each specialist nurse should be assigned to one or more neighbourhood services and have the commitment of her time to each service specified.
6 The principle should be adopted of introducing the nurse practitioner into primary health care.
7 The DHSS (now DOH) should agree a limited list of items and simple agents which may be prescribed by nurses as part of a nursing care programme, and issue guidelines to enable nurses to control drug dosage in well-defined circumstances.
8 To establish and be recognised as a primary health care team, each general medical practice and the community nurses associated with it should come to an understanding of the team's objectives and individuals' roles within it.

That understanding should be incorporated into a written agreement signed jointly by the practice partners and by the manager of the neighbourhood nursing service on behalf of the relevant health authority.

The agreement should name the doctors and community nurses

who together form the primary care team and should guarantee the right of the team members to be consulted on any changes proposed in its composition.

The making of such an agreement should be a qualifying condition for any incentive payments which may be introduced to improve quality in general practice (as suggested in the recent policy statement of the Royal College of General Practitioners).

9　The Government should invite the Health Advisory Service, with its established reputation, credibility and acceptance by the professions, to take on responsibility for identifying and promoting good practice in primary health care.

10　Subsidies to general practitioners enabling them to employ staff to perform nursing duties should be phased out.

11　Within two years the United Kingdom Central Council for Nursing, Midwifery and Health Visiting and the English National Board should introduce a common training course for all first-level nurses wishing to work outside hospital in what are now the fields of health visiting, district nursing and school nursing.

12　The provision of nursing services in the community should remain the responsibility of district health authorities. We would urge, however, that in due course the Government should give consideration to amalgamating family practitioner committees and district health authorities and so bring all primary health care services under the control of one body.

13　A short but thorough manpower planning exercise on a practical (as distinct from purely academic) basis should be undertaken to ensure that the training and supply of community nurses is, and remains at, the appropriate level. The study should be supported by the NHS Management Board as an essential task in reviewing the adequacy and consistency of Regional plans.

Appendix 6: Selected Material from the Child Development Programme

Reproduced by kind permission of the Early Childhood Development Unit, University of Bristol. The forms and cartoons on the following pages are copyright and may not be reproduced without the permission of the Unit.

SAMPLE PROVIDER SUB-CONTRACT FOR CHILD DEVELOPMENT PROGRAMME COMPONENT OF HEALTH VISITING SERVICE

Aims

The Programme will target parents with a home visiting programme based on structural support methods, in order to:

a. Improve the quality of parenting and the health and overall development of the children of first-time parents;

b. Concentrate resources on this group so that their care of subsequent children will be improved;

c. Support parents with two or more children, who face problems in rearing them and maintaining their health and development;

d. Foster parental independence so that more constructive use is made of the services;

e. Where appropriate, make use of resources from the community to aid in that task.

The programme will take place in the context of the Health Authority/ Board/Trust policy and strategies, and in accordance with the principles of the 1989 Children Act and other policies aimed at fostering the role and responsibilities of parents.

1. Objectives

1.1 To use the principles and strategies of the Child Development Programme in supporting parents and encouraging the development of their child rearing competence.

1.2 To foster in the parents a sense of independence and control over their lives.

1.3 To facilitate the parents' use of the health service and their access to other services.

1.4 To help prevent specific infectious diseases by achieving as a minimum goal the highest immunisation targets set by the Department of Health and by the Health Authority/Board/Trust itself.

1.5 To implement the use of the Early Health and Development Monitor (EHDM) in order to monitor the effectiveness of all health visiting to parents and young children throughout the Authority/Board/Trust, as well as to evaluate the effectiveness of the Child Development Programme (CDP) component within the programme areas.

1.6 To undertake regular audits of the CDP, using:

    a. management and peer group review;

    b. the responses of parents, GPs, health and other professionals,

    c. information obtained from the EHD Monitor.

2. Description of the programme

2.1 Ante-natal programme visits will be made to all first-time patients in the target areas, to familiarise the visitor with the parents' overall situation, to give the parents the opportunity to get to know the visitor and to help them to understand the broad goals of the programme.

2.2 Monthly programme visits will be made after the birth to all families in the targeted areas or GP practices, starting at 11 days post-natally; these will continue for at least eight months for all first-time mothers, and for as long as is judged necessary for parents with two or more children; visiting beyond eight months for selected first-time mothers will continue for up to 16, 24 or 36 months, depending on the level of need; fathers will be involved in this programme as fully as possible.

2.3 These visits will take place according to the protocol of the Child

Development Programme, using the progress form and other resources such as cartoons to ensure maximum benefit from the programme.

2.4   Regular monthly checks (by questioning the parents) will be carried out on the hearing of all programme children, and steps will be taken to ensure attendance at the formal hearing test at the prescribed age of eight or nine months.

2.5   All programme parents will be encouraged to bring in their children for the regular developmental screening assessments undertaken in the GP surgeries or clinics.

2.6   First Parent Visitors (FPVs) and Family Visitors will provide accompanied visits for health visitor and other students.

3.   Population served

3.1   The programme will cover either selected target areas or GP practice areas, chosen on the basis of socio-economic and other criteria, or will cover the whole Authority.

3.2   Within these target areas, all first-time pregnant women and their partners, and selected parents with two or more children, will receive the programme.

3.3   The health and development of the children of all the parents defined in 3.1 and 3.2 will be the prime concern of the Programme.

4.   Location and staffing

4.1   The CDP visiting programme will be fully home-based; however the parents will be encouraged by programme visitors to make optimal use of the other services in the clinics/health centres or in the wider community.

4.2   Programme visiting will be undertaken:

   a.   By health visitors specially appointed for this work and trained and qualified as First Parent Visitors (FPVs);

   b.   By health visitor colleagues of the FPVs, known as Family Visitors, provided that they too are properly trained and willing to visit a specified minimum of at least ten selected families on an ongoing basis;

   c.   By other people in the same community as those they visit, provided they are selected, properly trained and monitored by health visitors, and provided the limits of their non-professional role are clearly defined and agreed.

4.3   The First Parent Visitors will not undertake any activities outside of the home visiting to first-time parents; their Family Visitor colleagues will do any needed normal (non-programme) visiting to families with two or more children, or to older first-time parents for whom the programme visiting has ended.

5.   Maintenance of standards, monitoring of effectiveness

5.1   Health visitors will act at all times in accordance with the Code of Professional Conduct of the United Kingdom Central Council for Nurses, Midwives and Health Visitors.

5.2   All programme visitors will be trained to a standard required by the Early Childhood Development Unit at the University of Bristol; the certification of FPVs will be undertaken by the Unit at regular intervals, in close consultation with the Management of the Authority/Board/Trust.

5.3   All visits to homes will be made by appointment, other than in exceptional circumstances, and fall-back provisions will be instituted to take account of unexpected breakdowns in these arrangements.

5.4   Referral will be made to other professionals or agencies whenever necessary to ensure child protection or the investigation and treatment of suspected illness or disabilities in a child or adult.

5.5   When the Early Health and Development Monitor has been introduced into the Authority, this will be completed on all families at the appropriate ages, and the Monitor cards sent in for coding.

5.6   Information obtained from the Monitor will be made directly accessible to individual health visitors, their managers, general practitioners, managers of the Authority/Board/Trust and other health professionals, providing them with health and development profiles or analyses relevant to their role and interests.

5.7   Quality assurance procedures will be established by the Early Childhood Development Unit (ECDU) for those involved in the programme, to enable the First Parent Visitors, the FPVT and the NOC to ensure the maintenance of standards of programme visiting and the effectiveness of the administrative structure.

6. Management of the programme

6.1 *First Parent Visitor Trainer*

6.11   At the end of the main training period for First Parent Visitors, one or more First Parent Visitor Trainers (FPVTs) will be selected and given appropriate training by the ECDU trainers, to enable the FPVTs to take responsibility for providing further training within the Authority/Board/Trust; FPVTs will need to have had at least one year's full-time training and experience as a first parent visitor, before selection as a trainer.

6.12   The FPVT will work in close collaboration with and under the guidance of the Authority's Nursing Officer Coordinator for the programme.

6.13   The FPVT will be allocated between 10 and 20% of her/his time for the training of programme visitors and for dissemination work aimed at expanding the programme within the Authority/Board/Trust; the trainer will retain between 80 and 90% of a normal First Parent Visitor caseload.

6.14   The period of appointment of an FPVT will normally be three years.

6.2 *Nursing Officer Co-ordinator*

6.21   A Senior Nurse will have responsibility as Nursing Officer Coordinator for the management of the programme, with primary responsibility for administration and oversight of the programme within the Authority/Board/Trust; if the population or area covered is large, there may be two or more Nursing Officer Coordinators.

6.22   The Nursing Officer Coordinator (N.O.C.) will normally chair the ongoing training seminars, assisted by the FPV Trainer. The N.O.C. will have oversight of the training programme, in support of the work of the FPV Trainer.

6.23   The N.O.C. will operate in close collaboration with the FPV Trainer in dissemination work aimed at expanding the programme within the Authority.

7. Training

7.1   The Early Childhood Development Unit (ECDU) will provide the initial training for the programme, according to the protocol set out in the programme documentation.

7.2 In the second year of programme operation a First Parent Visitor Trainer will be selected, in joint discussion and agreement between the N.O.C. and the ECDU; the FPVT will be trained by the ECDU in the second and third years. If an FPVT leaves her post, her/his replacement will be selected and trained by the Unit according to an agreed schedule.

7.3 After the three years of programme training by the ECDU, this Unit will, in association with the Authority/Board/Trust, monitor the quality of the training and the maintenance of programme standards.

7.4 The N.O.C. will receive appropriate guidance from the ECDU in regard to programme strategies, and, if desired, will be trained to do programme visiting to between five and ten families for six months. In subsequent years she will continue to administer the programme, monitor progress and support the work of the FPV Trainer.

7.5 If an FPV Trainer leaves an Authority or is promoted to a management position, the ECDU training team will be asked to provide her replacement with appropriate training as an FPV Trainer for at least one year, and at the end of that year to validate the quality of her work and insights into the Programme principles and strategies.

R4

Child's Progress

CONFIDENTIAL

Child's first name only ....

Date of visit [| | |]   Visitor [|]   Child's Code No. [|]

Note: Coding below refers to period since last visit

Fill in developmental card (ask M to describe C achievements in past month)

PROGRAMME IDEAS FROM PREVIOUS VISIT

Has M taken up and carried out new ideas discussed between you
during previous visit? (regardless of success or otherwise
of ideas) (N.B. NOT a rating of C's attainment)

Health	NAA	YVM
Language	NAA	YVM
Social	NAA	YVM
Cognitive	NAA	YVM
Nutritionl	NAA	YVM
Educationl	NAA	YVM
General	NAA	YVM

Is there an awareness of Child's present developmental needs?

NAA [YVM]

NEW IDEAS INITIATED
BY MOTHER RECENTLY
(which might help others)

a. _____

_____

b. _____

_____

_____

c. _____

_____

REVIEW OF DIET/SNACKS/DRINKS/SWEETS FOR C YESTERDAY

Breakfast	Mid-morning	Lunch	Mid-afternoon	Supper	Bed-time
....	....	....	....	....	....
....	....	....	....	....	....
		....		....	

MOTHER'S DIET (OPTIONAL)

....	....	....	....	....	....
....	....	....	....	....	....

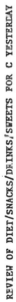

HEALTH SERVICE   G.P. or Consultant: Non-immun. visits ☐

No. of clinic
visits by M ☐   In-patient
                      hosp.(days) ☐   Medication:

Immunisation notes:
                      Out-patient
                      hosp. attendances ☐   ....

....

Reason for hosp. visits ....

Any supplementation?   Vitamins: ....   Minerals: ....

HOME HEALTH CONCERNS

Upper Resp./ENT:..................   Lower Resp./Chest ....

Digestive:..............   Skin:..............   Allergies:..............

Infectious diseases: ....   Other ills: ....   Accidents: ....

Emotional: ....   Other: ....   Hearing***: ....

Teeth problems: ....   *** ASK SPECIFICALLY

Cartoons given and discussed at this stage   (New cartoons selected:)

NEW IDEAS TO BE ATTEMPTED
What new developmental ideas are going to be attempted in the coming month?

Health: ....

Language: ....

Social: ....

Cognitive: ....

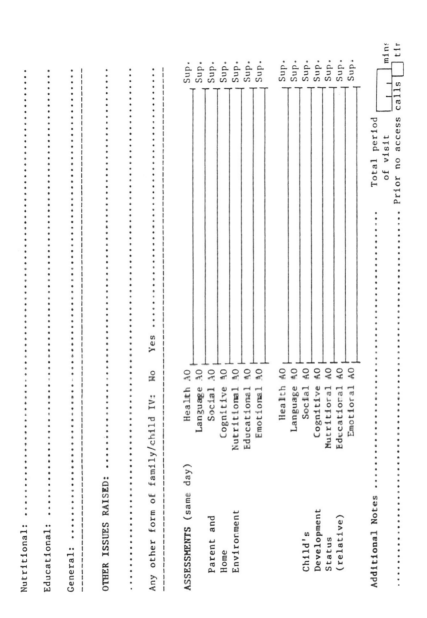

Nutritional: ....

Educational: ....

General: ....
|---------------------------------|

OTHER ISSUES RAISED: ....

....

Any other form of family/child IV: No   Yes ....
|---------------------------------|

ASSESSMENTS (same day)

Parent and Home Environment

Health   AO ————————————————— Sup.
Language   AO ————————————————— Sup.
Social   AO ————————————————— Sup.
Cognitive   AO ————————————————— Sup.
Nutritional AO ————————————————— Sup.
Educational AO ————————————————— Sup.
Emotional   AO ————————————————— Sup.

Child's Development Status (relative)

Health   AO ————————————————— Sup.
Language   AO ————————————————— Sup.
Social   AO ————————————————— Sup.
Cognitive   AO ————————————————— Sup.
Nutritional AO ————————————————— Sup.
Educational AO ————————————————— Sup.
Emotional   AO ————————————————— Sup.

Additional Notes ....

....

Total period of visit .... [ ] mins

Prior no access calls .... [ ] tir

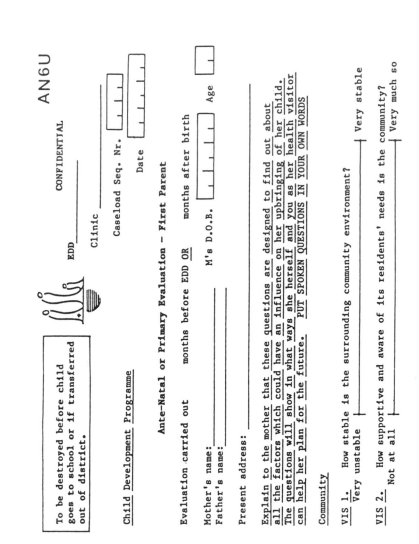

AN6U

To be destroyed before child
goes to school or if transferred
out of district.

EDD _____   CONFIDENTIAL

Clinic _____

Caseload Seq. Nr. [| |]

Date [| |]

Age [   ]

Child Development Programme

Ante-Natal or Primary Evaluation - First Parent

Evaluation carried out _____ months before EDD OR _____ months after birth

Mother's name: _____   M's D.O.B. [| |]
Father's name: _____

Present address: _____

Explain to the mother that these questions are designed to find out about
all the factors which could have an influence on her upbringing of her child.
The questions will show in what ways she herself and you as her health visitor
can help her plan for the future.   PUT SPOKEN QUESTIONS IN YOUR OWN WORDS

Community

VIS 1.   How stable is the surrounding community environment?
Very unstable |—————————————————————| Very stable

VIS 2.   How supportive and aware of its residents' needs is the community?
Not at all |—————————————————————| Very much so

Housing

VIS 11. Is M's accommodation (circle one or more):

Authy.   Priv.   M/F name   Grandp.   Grandp.   Others   Self   Shared   Only   Other accom
Rented   Rented   rents   owns   own   Owned   w.others temp   promised

VIS 12. Quality of accommodation:
         Very limited ├────────────────────────────────────┤ Top quality

M 14. Are you crowded here at home? (Take a/c space, adults, children, C's ages)

       Very crowded ├────────────────────────────────────┤ No crowding

M 15. How close are you to private and safe play space for children?
       Very far off ├────────────────────────────────────┤ Very close by

M 16. Have you plans to: Stay where   Apply for other   Move   Move
                             you are   accommodatn   shortly   later

VIS 17. Minimum necessary action on housing.
         None   M to apply   V contact Housing   V contact Social   V act self

Health Environment

M 21. How adequate is the heating here, especially in the baby's room.
       NAA ├────────────────────────────────────┤ VSI

M 22. Do you think there is dampness or mould in the home?
       NAA ├────────────────────────────────────┤ YVM

M 23. Do you or others in this home consider that anything can be done about
       the heating or dampness? ____

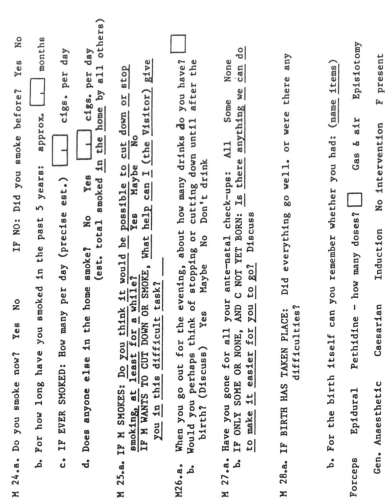

M 24.a. Do you smoke now? Yes No   IF NO: Did you smoke before? Yes No

b. For how long have you smoked in the past 5 years: approx. [   ] months

c. IF EVER SMOKED: How many per day (precise est.) [   ] cigs. per day

d. Does anyone else in the home smoke? No Yes [   ] cigs. per day
(est. total smoked in the home by all others)

M 25.a. IF M SMOKES: Do you think it would be possible to cut down or stop
smoking, at least for a while?   Yes Maybe No
IF M WANTS TO CUT DOWN OR SMOKE, What help can I (the Visitor) give
you in this difficult task? _____

M26.a. When you go out for the evening, about how many drinks do you have?
b. Would you perhaps think of stopping or cutting down until after the
birth? (Discuss) Yes Maybe No Don't drink

M 27.a. Have you gone for all your ante-natal check-ups: All Some None
b. IF ONLY SOME OR NONE, AND C NOT YET BORN: Is there anything we can do
to make it easier for you to go? Discuss

POST M 28.a. IF BIRTH HAS TAKEN PLACE: Did everything go well, or were there any
difficulties?

b. For the birth itself can you remember whether you had: (name items)

Forceps Epidural Pethidine - how many doses? [   ] Gas & air Episiotomy

Gen. Anaesthetic Caesarian Induction No intervention F present

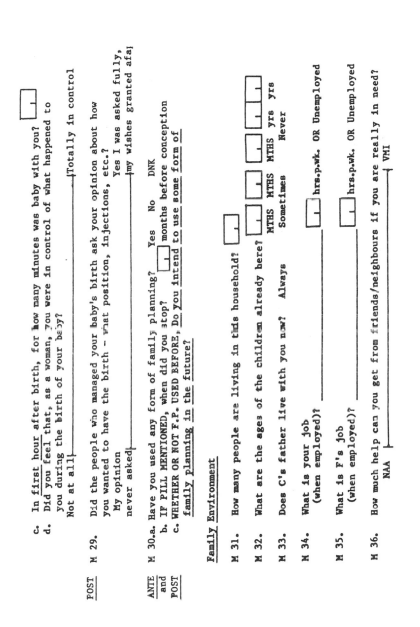

c. In first hour after birth, for how many minutes was baby with you? ☐

d. Did you feel that, as a woman, you were in control of what happened to you during the birth of your baby?

Not at all |_____| Totally in control

POST

M 29. Did the people who managed your baby's birth ask your opinion about how you wanted to have the birth – what position, injections, etc.?

My opinion   Yes I was asked fully,

never asked |_____| my wishes granted afap

ANTE
and
POST

M 30.a. Have you used any form of family planning?   Yes   No   DNK

b. IF PILL MENTIONED, when did you stop? ☐ months before conception

c. WHETHER OR NOT F.P. USED BEFORE, Do you intend to use some form of family planning in the future?

Family Environment

M 31. How many people are living in this household? ☐

M 32. What are the ages of the children already here? ☐ ☐ ☐

MTHS MTHS MTHS yrs yrs

M 33. Does C's father live with you now?   Always   Sometimes   Never

M 34. What is your job
(when employed)? _____ ☐ hrs.p.wk. OR Unemployed

M 35. What is F's job
(when employed)? _____ ☐ hrs.p.wk. OR Unemployed

M 36. How much help can you get from friends/neighbours if you are really in need?

NAA |_____| VMI

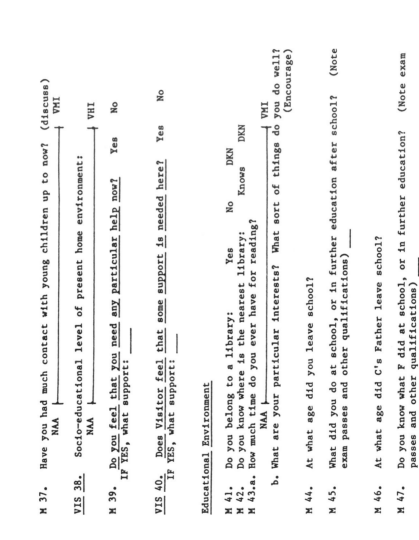

M 37.   Have you had much contact with young children up to now?   (discuss)
      NAA ⊢————————┤ VMI

VIS 38.   Socio-educational level of present home environment:
      NAA ⊢————————┤ VHI

M 39.   <u>Do you feel that you need any particular help now?</u>   Yes   No
      IF YES, what support: _____

VIS 40.   <u>Does Visitor feel that some support is needed here?</u>   Yes   No
      IF YES, what support: _____

Educational Environment

M 41.   Do you belong to a library: Yes   No   DKN
M 42.   Do you know where is the nearest library: Knows   DKN
M 43.a.   How much time do you ever have for reading?
      NAA ⊢————————┤ VMI
   b. What are your particular interests?   What sort of things do you do well?
                                               (Encourage)

M 44.   At what age did you leave school?

M 45.   What did you do at school, or in further education after school?   (Note
      exam passes and other qualifications) _____

M 46.   At what age did C's Father leave school?

M 47.   Do you know what F did at school, or in further education?   (Note exam
      passes and other qualifications) _____

VIS 48.a. Estimate of LTYM

Abs. [————————————————] Pres.

b. Books in the home?

Abs. [————————————————] Pres.

VIS 49. Has anything been suggested in regard to LTYM or library or other educational issues?

Mother's Health

M 51.a. How well do you feel in yourself now? (Mark A for Ante, P for Post-Natal)

NAA well [————————————————] Very well

ANTE and POST

b. Are you on any particular tablets at the moment? Yes No

IF YES: which ones? ___ what are they for? ___

M 52.a. Have you been pregnant before this occasion? Yes No

b. IF YES: Could you tell me what happened before?

1. 2. 3. 4.

M 53. Do you feel tired most of the time?

NAA [————————————————] YVM

Do you often feel miserable or depressed?

NAA [————————————————] YVM

Do you often have bad headaches?

NAA [————————————————] YVM

Are there times when you don't want to go out or meet people? Often

NAA [————————————————] YVM

M 54.   (PUT INTO OWN WORDS)   When you think about your life, about the good things and the bad things in it, would you say that most of what has happened to you has happened because of good luck and bad luck, that people are just not appreciated for what they try to do, and that it's not worth planning things. How much of what has happened to you in life is due to outside factors, and how much to things in your control.   (Discuss, then estimate.)

Due to out-   All in my
side factors   ⊢————————————————————————⊣   own control

<u>VIS</u> 55.a. Estimate level of low s.e:

    Normal ⊢————————————————⊣ VLOW

  <u>b.</u> Estimate level of d/d:
    O(NAA) ⊢————————————————⊣ VM

  <u>c.</u> Estimate ps:
    O(NAA) ⊢————————————————⊣ VRGD

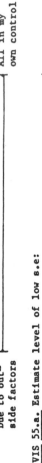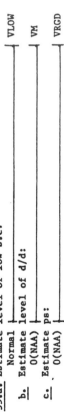

M 56.   Have you changed your diet or do you plan to change your diet to take into account your pregnancy (or the birth)?   Yes   Not sure   No

<u>VIS</u> <u>57.</u>   Discuss M's diet. (ask re prev.day; check if this pattern general)
    V.poor ⊢————————————————⊣V.good

<u>VIS</u> <u>58.</u>   What does M (<u>and/or the Visitor</u>) think can be done <u>to overcome or minimise any of the health problems identified here such as</u> M's <u>general feeling of ill health, low s.e. or feeling of d/d.</u>

<u>VIS</u> <u>59.</u>   If the crude preliminary dietary assessment above indicate <u>a diet that is poor or only moderate,</u> will M be shown <u>how to carry out a weighed intake prior to a formal assessment and recommendations?</u>
    Yes   No   M unwilling

M 60 a. Have you thought about how you are going to feed the baby?

V.hostile to b.fdg ├──────────────────────────────────┤ V.keen on it

b. Discuss advantages of br. fdg. but recognise M's freedom of choice

Life Stresses

M 61. Is there someone in whom you can really confide, whom you can talk to about your trials and troubles?

NAA ├──────────────────────────────────┤ Can confide totally

M 62. Are your own parents (OR adoptive parents) alive? (Incl. step-parent if regarded as own parent). IF NOT, how old were you when they died?

Mother alive   Mother died when M ☐ years old   Father alive   Father died when M ☐ years old

M 63. Just to make sure how much financial and other support you will have when the baby arrives, could you tell me about C's father. Are you:

Married   Planning marr.   Not yet sure   Separated   Planning sep.

M 64. Have there been any serious and unexpected worries or problems in your life over the past few years, which might make it difficult for you to cope with bringing up your new child?   Yes   No

IF YES: how serious were these problems?

NAA ├──────────────────────────────────┤ Very serious

M 65. Is there anything that you or I can do, or my colleagues, to help you overcome any problems that you may still have?

Thank you for being so helpful in answering these questions. It has shown what you and I can do to try to make things easier for you as a new mother.

Pregnant Mothers: what to eat?

Child Development Project

N22

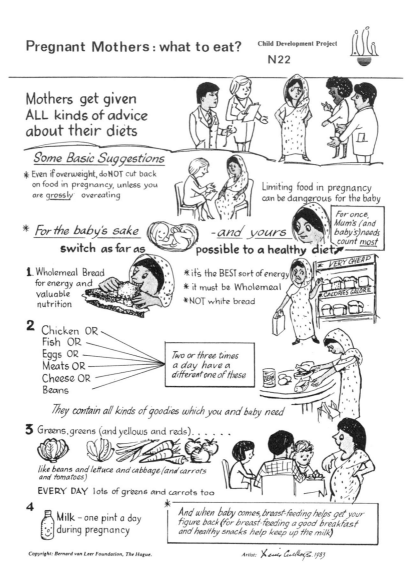

Mothers get given
ALL kinds of advice
about their diets

Some Basic Suggestions

* Even if overweight, do NOT cut back
  on food in pregnancy, unless you
  are grossly overeating

Limiting food in pregnancy
can be dangerous for the baby

* *For the baby's sake*   *— and yours*

For once,
Mum's (and
baby's) needs
count most

switch as far as   possible to a healthy diet

1. Wholemeal Bread
   for energy and
   valuable
   nutrition

* it's the BEST sort of energy
* it must be Wholemeal
* NOT white bread

VERY CHEAP

CALORIES GALORE

2 Chicken OR
  Fish OR
  Eggs OR
  Meats OR
  Cheese OR
  Beans

Two or three times
a day have a
different one of these

They contain all kinds of goodies which you and baby need

3 Greens, greens (and yellows and reds) . . . . . .

like beans and lettuce and cabbage (and carrots
and tomatoes)

EVERY DAY lots of greens and carrots too

4 Milk – one pint a day
  during pregnancy

*And when baby comes, breast-feeding helps get your
figure back (for breast-feeding a good breakfast
and healthy snacks help keep up the milk)*

Copyright: Bernard van Leer Foundation, The Hague.

Artist: *Leslie Culley* 1983

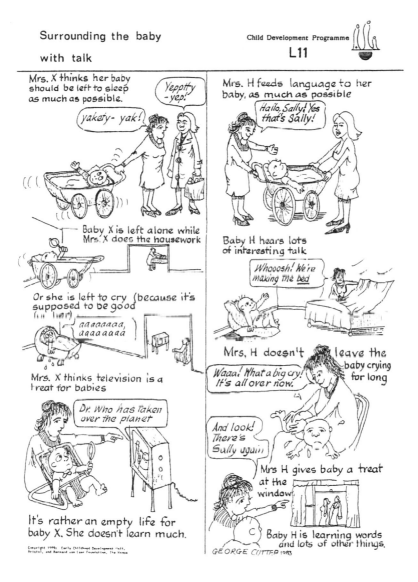

Surrounding the baby with talk

Child Development Programme
L11

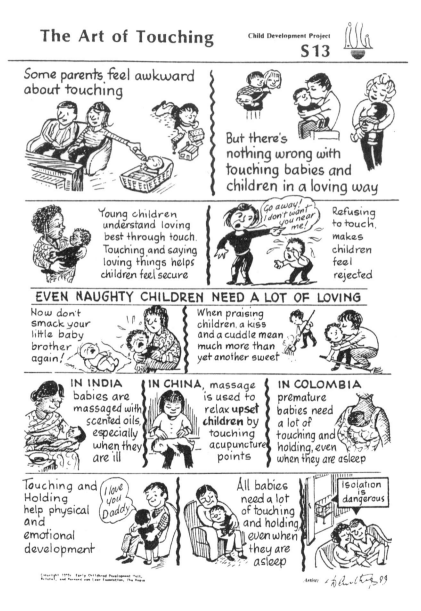

The Art of Touching

Child Development Project

S 13

Some parents feel awkward about touching

But there's nothing wrong with touching babies and children in a loving way

Young children understand loving best through touch. Touching and saying loving things helps children feel secure

Go away! I don't want you near me!

Refusing to touch, makes children feel rejected

EVEN NAUGHTY CHILDREN NEED A LOT OF LOVING

Now don't smack your little baby brother again!

When praising children, a kiss and a cuddle mean much more than yet another sweet

IN INDIA babies are massaged with scented oils, especially when they are ill

IN CHINA, massage is used to relax **upset children** by touching acupuncture points

IN COLOMBIA premature babies need a lot of touching and holding, even when they are asleep

Touching and Holding help physical and emotional development

I love you Daddy

All babies need a lot of touching and holding, even when they are asleep

Isolation is dangerous

THE LIBRARY

Dungeon or Delight?

Child Development Project

E3A

Copyright: Bernard van Leer Foundation, The Hague.

Artist: Denis Curthoys 1983

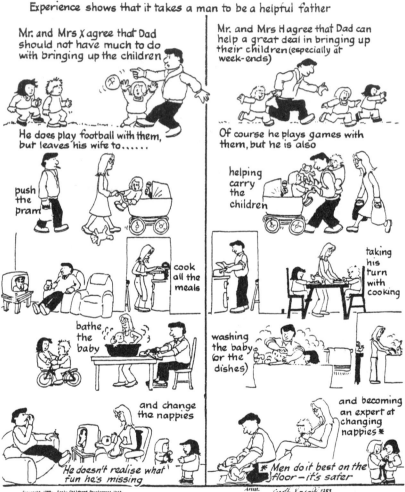

Today's Fathers are Tough

Child Development Programme

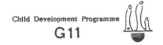

G11

Experience shows that it takes a man to be a helpful father

Mr. and Mrs X agree that Dad should not have much to do with bringing up the children

Mr. and Mrs H agree that Dad can help a great deal in bringing up their children (especially at week-ends)

He does play football with them, but leaves his wife to......

Of course he plays games with them, but he is also

push the pram

helping carry the children

cook all the meals

taking his turn with cooking

bathe the baby

washing the baby (or the dishes)

and change the nappies

and becoming an expert at changing nappies *

He doesn't realise what fun he's missing

* Men do it best on the floor — it's safer

Copyright 1989: Early Childhood Development Unit, Bristol, and Bernard van Leer Foundation, The Hague

Artist. *Geoff Lapaire* 1989

Sweet at sixteen?

Child Development Project

H 8

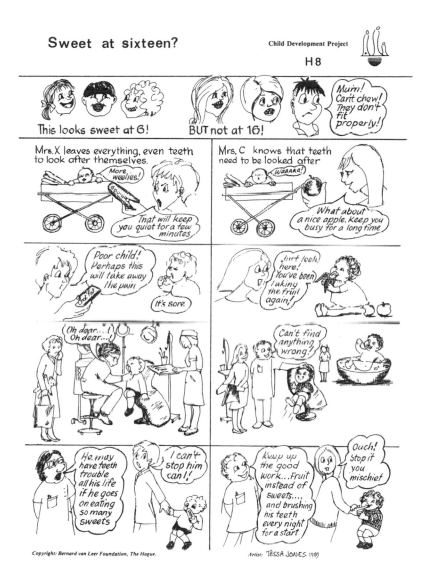

Copyright: Bernard van Leer Foundation, The Hague.

Artist: TESSA JONES 1983

References and Further Reading

Acheson R.M. & Hall D.J. (1976) Epilogue. In Acheson R., Hall D. & Aird L. (eds.) *Seminars in Community Medicine*. Oxford University Press, Oxford.

Adelstein A.M. (1976) Indicators of need, demand and use. In Acheson R., Hall D. & Aird L. (eds.) *Seminars in Community Medicine*. Oxford University Press, Oxford.

Alderman C. (1989) Evaluating the Quality of Care. *Nursing Standard* 4(4), 1-3.

Anderson E. *et al.* (1978) *Development and Implementation of Curriculum Model for Community Nurse Practitioners*. United States Department of Health Education and Welfare, University of Texas, Houston.

Arstein S. (1969) A ladder of citizen participation. *Journal of the American Institute of Planners* (July), 214-19.

Ashton J. & Seymour H. (1985) An approach to health promotion in one region. *Community Medicine*, **7**, 78-86.

Ashton J., Grey P. & Barnard K. (1986) Healthy Cities – WHO's new public health initiative. *Health Promotion*, **1**(3), 319-24.

Ashton J & Seymour H. (1988) *The New Public Health*. Open University Press, Milton Keynes.

Bagust A., Prescott J. & Smith A. (1988) *Nursing manpower project final report*, NWRHA, Manchester.

Barber B. & Scholes M. (1979) Learning to live with computers. *Nursing Mirror*, **149**(1), 22-4.

Barclay Report (1982) *Social Workers: Their Role and Tasks*. National Institute for Social Work, Bedford Press, London.

Barker W. (1984) *Child Development Programme*. Early Childhood Development Unit, Senate House, University of Bristol, Bristol.

Barker W. & Anderson R. (1988) *Child Development Programme: An Evaluation of Process and Outcomes*. Early Child Development Unit, University of Bristol.

Barnard P.J., Hammon N.V., Morton J., Long J.B. & Clark I.A. (1981) Consistency and compatibility in human computer dialogue. *International Journal of Man Machine Studies*, **15**, 87-134.

Baron R.A. (1986) *Behaviour in organisations: understanding and managing the human side of work*: 2nd edn, Allyn & Bacon, Boston.

Barr L. & Moores B. (1982) Nurse-patient dependency revisited. *Journal of Advanced Nursing*, **7**, 269-72.

Bayley M. (1982) Community care and the elderly. In Glendenning F. (ed.) *Care in the Community: Recent Research and Current Projects*. Beth Johnston Foundation Publication in association with Department of Adult Education, University of Keele, England.

Becker H. (1967) Whose side are we on? *Social Problems* **14**, 241.

Belfast Areas of Special Social Needs (1976) A Report by the Project Team Belfast, HMSO.

Benson J. (1976) The concept of community. In Timms N. & Watson D. (eds.) *Talking about Welfare*. Routledge & Kegan Paul, London.

Berg H.V. (1974) Nursing audit and outcome criteria. *Nursing Clinics of North America* **9**(2), 331–5.

Berger P.L. (1965) Towards a sociological understanding of psychoanalysis. *Social Research* **36**, (Spring).

Bergman R. (1981) *Where do we go from here?* Paper presented at Conference Primary Health Care in Europe: The Role of the Health Visitor, North East London Polytechnic, London.

Bernard J. (1973) My four resolutions: an autobiographical history of the A.S.A. In Huber J. (ed.) *Changing Women in a Changing Society*. University of Chicago Press, Chicago.

Billingham K. (1991) Public health and the community. *Health Visitor*, **64**(2), 40–3.

Blane, D. (1989) Preventive Medicine and Public Health. In *Readings for a New Public Health* (ed. by J. Martin and D. McQueen). University of Edinburgh Press, Edinburgh.

Blattner B. (1981) *Holistic Nursing*. Prentice Hall, New Jersey.

Bloch D. (1975) Evaluation of nursing care in terms of process and outcome. Issues in research and quality assurance. *Nursing Research* **24**(4), 256–63.

Bowman M.P. (1986) *Nursing Management and Education: a conceptual approach to change*. Croom Helm, London.

Bradshaw J. (1972) The concept of social need. *New Society* **30**, 640–3.

Brighton Women and Science Group (1980) *Alice Through the Microscope*. Virago, London.

Buchan D.A. & Boddy D. (1983) Advanced Technology and the Quality of Working Life: the effects of computerized controls on biscuit making, *J. Occ. Psychology*, **56**, 109–19.

Bucher R. & Strauss A.L. (1961) Professions in process. *American Journal of Sociology* **66**, 325–34.

Butcher H., Collis P., Glen A. & Sills P. (1980) *Community Groups in Action: Case Studies and Analysis*. Routledge & Kegan Paul, London.

Buxton M., Packwood T. & Keen J. (1989) *Resource Management processes and progress – monitoring the six hospital pilot sites*, HMSO, London.

Campbell A., Converse P. & Rodgers W. (1976) *The Quality of American Life: Perceptions, Evaluations and Satisfaction*. Sage, New York.

Carlisle E. (1972) The conceptual structure of social indicators. In Schonfield A. & Shaw S. (eds.) *Social Indicators and Social Policy*. Heinemann, London.

Carpenter M. (1977) The New Managerialism and Professionalism in Nursing. In

Health and the Division of Labour (Ed. by M. Stacey, M. Reid, C. Heath and R. Dingwall). Churchill Livingstone, Edinburgh.

Central Advisory Council for Education in England (1967) Children and their primary schools. *The Plowden Report*, HMSO, London.

Chalmers K.I. & Luker K.A. (1991) The Development of the Health Visitor-Client Relationship. *Scandinavian Journal of Caring Sciences* **5**(1), 33–41.

Chen M.M., Bush J.W. & Patrick D.L. (1975) Social indicators for health planning and policy analysis. *Policy Sciences* **6**, 71–89.

Clark D.B. (1973) The concept of community: a re-examination. Republished (1981) in Henderson P. & Thomas D. (eds.) *Readings in Community Work*. Allen & Unwin, London.

Clark J. (1973) *A Family Visitor*. Royal College of Nursing, London.

Clark J. (1980) A framework for health visiting. *Health Visitor* **53**(10), 418–20.

Clarke D. (1986) Showing that it can be done. *Health Service Journal*, 96, (5019); 1297.

Colliére M.F. (1980) Development of primary health care. *International Nursing Review* **27**(6), 169–72.

Colliére M.F. (1981) *The Role of the Health Visitor*. Paper presented at conference: Primary Health Care in Europe: The role of the Health Visitor. North East London Polytechnic, London.

Colliety P. (1988) An Evaluation of the Health Visiting Process (part one). *Senior Nurse* Vol. 8, No. 12, 13–18.

Colliety P. (1989) An Evaluation of the Health Visiting Process (part two). *Senior Nurse* Vol. 9, No. 1, 13–16.

Comer L. (1974) *Wedlocked Women*. Leeds Feminist Books, Leeds.

Community Projects Foundation (1982) *Community Development Towards a National Perspective. The Work of Community Projects Foundation 1978–1982*. Community Projects Foundation, London.

Coombs R. & Cooper D. (1990) *Accounting for Patients? Information Technology and the implementation of the N.H.S. white paper*, PICT Publications n10, Oxford.

Council for the Education and Training of Health Visitors (1976) *The Health Visitor: Functions and Implications for Training*. Council for the Education and Training of Health Visitors, London.

Council for the Education and Training of Health Visitors (1977) *An Investigation into the Principles of Health Visiting*. Council for the Education and Training of Health Visitors, London.

Council for the Education and Training of Health Visitors (1982a) *Health Visiting Principles in Practice*. Council for the Education and Training of Health Visitors, London.

Council for the Education and Training of Health Visitors (1982b) *Time to Learn*. A report of Standing Conference of representatives of health visitor education and training centres working group on the content and length of the health visitor course. Council for the Education and Training of Health Visitors, London.

Cowie S. (1991) *The Teamwork Nursing System – care in the community*,

NWRHA, Manchester.

Creasy D. (1987) Korner related computer systems. *Health Service Journal*, **97** (5039), 8–9.

Cumberlege Report (1986) Report of the community nursing review. *Neighbourhood Nursing*, A focus for care, HMSO, London.

Data Protection Act (1989a) *Guideline 1: Introduction to the Art*, Data Protection Registrar, Wilmslow.

Data Protection Act (1989b) *Guideline 4: The data protection principles*. Data Protection Registrar, Wilmslow.

Dearlove J. (1974) The control of change and the regulation of community action. In Jones D. & Mayo M. (eds.) *Community Work One*. Routledge & Kegan Paul, London.

Denniss G. & Wickstead D.P. (1984) *Chalkhill Neighbourhood Project*. Personnel Communication, London.

Department of the Environment (1981) *Census Information Note Number 2: Urban Deprivation Inner Cities Directorate*. HMSO, London.

Department of Health (1989a) *Working for Patients*. HMSO, London.

Department of Health (1989b) *Promoting Better Health*. HMSO, London.

Department of Health (1989c) *Caring for people, community care in the next decade and beyond*. HMSO, London.

Department of Health (1990) *Working for Patients – Framework for information systems; Information* (Annex 5) Report of the Project 34 Working Group on community health services. HMSO, London.

Department of Health (1990) *Working for Patients – Framework for information systems, overview* (Working Paper 11). HMSO, London.

Department of Health (1990) *Working for Patients – Framework for information systems; the next steps*. HMSO, London.

Department of Health (1991a) *The Health of the Nation*. A Consultative Document for Health in England. HMSO, London.

Department of Health (1991b) *Care management and assessment summary of practice guidelines*. HMSO, London.

Department of Health and Personal Social Sciences (1990) Statistics for England.

Department of Health and Social Security (1972) *Management arrangements for the reorganised NHS*. HMSO, London.

Department of Health and Social Security (1976) *Report on the Committee on Child Health Services; Fit for the Future*. HMSO, London.

Department of Health and Social Security (1979) *Report of the Royal Commission on the NHS* (Chairman Sir Alec Merrison). HMSO, London.

Department of Health and Social Security (1980) *Inequalities in Health: Report of a Research Working Group*. (Known as the Black Report) HMSO, London.

Department of Health and Social Security (1982) *First report of the steering group on health services information* (Chairman Mrs Edith Korner) The collection and use of information about hospital clinical activity. HMSO, London.

Department of Health and Social Security (1983a) *Steering Group on Health*

Services Information. A report from a working group on Community Health Services.

Department of Health and Social Security (1983b) *NHS management inquiry* (Chairman Sir Roy Griffiths). HMSO, London.

Department of Health and Social Security (1984) *Second report of the steering group on health services information* (Chairman Mrs Edith Korner) The collection and use of information about patient transport services. HMSO, London.

Department of Health and Social Security (1984) *Third report of the steering group on health services information* (Chairman Mrs Edith Korner) The collection and use of information about health services manpower. HMSO, London.

Department of Health and Social Security (1984) *Fourth report of the steering group on health services information* (Chairman Mrs Edith Korner) The collection and use of information about activity in hospitals and the community. HMSO, London.

Department of Health and Social Security (1985) *Fifth Report of the steering group on health services information* (Chairman Mrs Edith Korner) The collection and use of information about services for and in the community. HMSO, London.

Department of Health and Social Security (1985) *Sixth report of the steering group on health services information* (Chairman Mrs Edith Korner) The collection and use of information about health services finance. HMSO, London.

Department of Health and Social Security (1986) *Nurse demand methods – whither now?* Report of the NHS operational research service on nurse staffing methodologies. HMSO, London.

Department of Health and Social Security (1986) *Resource management in health authorities* HN (86) 34. HMSO, London.

Derrybery M. (1939) Nursing accomplishments as revealed by case records. *Public Health Report* **54**, 20–35.

Dickoff J., James P. & Wiedenback E. (1968) Theory in a practice discipline. *Nursing Research* **17**(5), 415–35.

Dingwall R. (1976) The social organisation of health visitor training I. The social theories of health visitors. *Nursing Times* **72**(7), 29–32.

Dingwall R. (1977) *The Social Organisation of Health Visitor Training.* Croom Helm, London.

Dingwall R., Eekelar J. & Murray T. (1983) *The protection of children: state intervention in family life.* Basil Blackwell, Oxford.

Donabedian A. (1969) Some issues in evaluating the quality of nursing care. *American Journal of Public Health* **59**(10); 1833–6.

Dowling S. (1983) *Health for a Change; The Provision of Preventive Health Care in Pregnancy and Early Childhood.* Child Poverty Action in association with the National Extension College, Cambridge.

Draper P. (1991) *Health through public policy.* Green Print, London.

Drennan V. (1984) *Paddington and Kensington Health District: Personal*

Communication. London. (Unpublished.)

Drennan V. (1986) Developments in health visiting. *Health Visitor*, **59**(4), 108-110.

Drennan V. (1988) *Health visitors and groups*. Heinemann Nursing, Oxford.

Du Bois B. (1983) Passionate scholarship: notes on values knowing and method of feminist social science. In Bowles G.B. & Duelli-Klein R. (eds.) *Theories of Women's Studies*. Routledge & Kegan Paul, London.

Dunnel K. & Dobbs J. (1983) *Nurses working in the Community* OPCS. HMSO, London.

Dylak P. (1991) *Analysis of a dependency driven nurse manpower planning system*. Unpublished M.Sc. Thesis, University of Manchester.

Edwards J. (1975) Social indicators; urban deprivation and positive discrimination. *Journal of Social Policy* **4**(3), 275-87.

Elliot H.C. (1974) Similarities and differences between science and commonsense. In Turner R. (ed.) *Ethnomethodology*. Penguin, Harmondsworth.

Epp J. (1986) *Achieving health for all: a framework for health promotion*. Department of Health and Welfare, Ottawa, Canada.

Etzioni A. (1964) *Modern Organisations*. Prentice Hall, Englewood Cliffs.

Fatchett A.B. (1990) Health visiting - a withering profession? *Journal of Advanced Nursing* **15**, 216-22.

Figlio K. (1982) How does illness mediate social relations? Workmen's compensation and medico-legal practices 1890 1940. In Wright & Treacher (ed.) *The Problem of Medical Knowledge*. Edinburgh University Press, Edinburgh.

Financial Information Project (1980) *First research report of the Financial Information Project*. HMSO, London.

Forder A. (1974) *Concepts in Social Administration*. Routledge & Kegan Paul, London.

Fox J. (1987) Artificial intelligence in the workplace. *Psychology at work*, 3rd edn (Ed. P.B. Warr). Penguin, Harmondsworth.

Freeman, R. (1990) Information - lifeblood of the NHS. *Health Service Journal* 100 (5190); 332-33.

Freidson E. (1975) *Profession of Medicine*. Dodd, Mead & Co., New York.

Freidson E. (1977) The future of professionalisation. In Stacey M., Reid M., Heath C. & Dingwall R. (eds.) *Health and the Division of Labour*. Croom Helm, London.

Friel P.B., Reznikoff M. & Rosenberg M. (1969) Attitudes toward computers amongst nursing personnel in a general hospital. *Connecticut Medicine* **33**(5); 307-8.

Friedman M. (1981) *Family nursing theory assessment*, 2nd edn. Appleton Century Press.

Fruin D.J. (1971) Analysis of need. In Brown M.J. (ed.) *Social Issues and Social Services*. Charles Knight, London.

Gault A.R. (1982) The Aberdeen formula as an illustration of the difficulty of determining nursing requirements. *International Journal of Nursing Studies* **19**(2); 61-77.

Gilbert N. (1972) Assessing Service - delivery methods. Some unsettled questions. *Welfare in Review* **10**(3), 25-33.

Gilmore M., Bruce N. & Hunt M. (1974) *The work of the Nursing Team in General Practice.* Council of the Education and Training of Health Visitors, London.

Glass N. (1976) The meaning of the term need. In Acheson R., Hall D. & Aird L. (eds.) *Seminars in Community Medicine.* Oxford University Press, Oxford.

Goldberg E.M., Mortimer A. & Williams B. (1970) *Helping the aged; a Field Experiment in Social Work.* Allen & Unwin, London.

Goeppinger J., Lassiter P. & Wilcox B. (1982) Community health in community competence. *Nursing Outlook* **30**(8), 464-7.

Goodwin S., Dunford H. & McNeil L. (1991) One year on - the effects on GP contracts. *Community Outlook,* May pp. 17-19.

Greer S. & Minar D. (1969) *The Concept of Community.* Aldine Press, Chicago.

Hancock T. & Duhl L. (1985) *Healthy Cities: Promoting Health in the Urban Context.* A background working paper for the healthy cities symposium. WHO, Copenhagen.

Handy C.B. (1988) *Understanding Organisations* Penguin, Harmondsworth.

Hatch S. & Sherratt R. (1973) Positive discrimination and the distribution of deprivations. *Policy and Politics* **1**(3), 223-40.

Henderson J. (1978) What do health visitors do? *Nursing Mirror* **147**(11), 20-32.

Henderson P. & Thomas D. (1980) *Skills in Neighbourhood Work.* Allen & Unwin, London.

Hicks D. (1976) *Primary Health Care.* HMSO, London.

Hillery G.A. (1955) Definition of community - areas of agreement. *Rural Sociology* **20** (June), 111-23.

Hilger E.E. (1974) Developing outcome criteria. *Nursing Clinics of North America* **9**(2), 323-9.

Hirsch F. (1977) *Social Limits to Growth.* Routledge & Kegan Paul, London.

Hobbs P. (1973) *Aptitude or Environment.* Royal College of Nursing, London.

Hodge R.W. & Klorman R. (1979) Dynamic social indicator models; some problems of theory concept and data. *Sociology and Social Research* **63**(4), 613-48.

House of Commons (1989) *The Children Act.* HMSO, London.

House of Commons (1990) *National Health Service and Community Care Bill.* HMSO, London.

Hoy D. (1990) Computer assisted nursing care planning in the UK. *Information Technology in Nursing* **2**(2); 22-3.

Hull W. (1989) Measuring Effectiveness in Health Visiting. *Health Visitor* **62**, 113-15.

Huntington J. (1981) *Social Work and General Medical Practice.* Allen & Unwin, London.

Imber V. (1977) *A Classification of the English Personal Social Service Authorities. Statistical and Research Series No. 16.* Department of Health and Social Security, London.

Jarman B. (1983) Identification of underprivileged areas. *British Medical Journal* **286**, 1705-9.

Jeffreys M. (1965) The uncertain health visitor. *New Society* **6**(161), 16-18.

Jones K., Brown J. & Bradshaw J. (1978) *Issues in Social Policy.* Routledge & Kegan Paul, London.

Karhausen L. (1978) Introduction. In Holland W.W. & Karhausen L. (eds.) *Health Care and Epidemiology,* p. 1. Henry Kimpton, London.

Kenner C. (1986) *Whose needs count?* Bedford Square Press, NCVO, London.

Kiernan, K. & Wicks, M. (1990), *Family Changes and full-time policy.* Family Policy Studies Centre, London.

Knight B. & Hayes R. (1981) *Self Help in the Inner City.* Voluntary Services Council, London.

Knox E.G. (1987) *Health Care Information.* Report of a joint working group of the Korner committee on health services information and the faculty of community medicine. Nuffield Trust, Oxford.

Konig R. (1968) *The Community.* Allen & Unwin, London.

Krampf, S. & Robinson S. (1984) Managing nurses' attitudes toward computers. *Nursing Management* **15**(7); 29–34.

Krupat E. & Guild W. (1980) Defining the city: The use of objective and subjective measures for community description. *Journal of Social Issues* **36**(3), 9–28.

Labonte R. (1986) Social inequality and health public policy. *Health Promotion,* **1**(3), 341–51.

Land K. & McMillen M. (1978) *Demographic Data and Social Indicators.* Paper presented at American Sociological Association, San Francisco, California.

Lave J.R. & Lave L.B. (1977) Measuring the effectiveness of prevention 1. *Milbank Memorial Fund Quarterly 'Health and Society'* (Spring), 273–89.

Lind G. & Wiseman C. (1980) Setting health priorities: a review of concepts and approaches. *Journal of Social Policy* **4**, 411–40.

Lindeman C.A. (1976a) Measuring quality of nursing care research procedures. *Journal of Nursing Administration* **6**(1), 7–9.

Lindeman C.A. (1976b) Measuring quality of nursing care review of current research projects. *Journal of Nursing Administration* **6**(2), 16–19.

Luker K.A. (1978) Goal attainment: a possible model for assessing the work of the health visitor. *Nursing Times* **75**(35), 1488–90.

Luker K.A. (1982a) *Evaluating Health Visiting Practice.* Royal College of Nursing, London.

Luker K.A. (1982b) An attempt at process outcome evaluation. *British Journal of Geriatric Nursing* **2**(1), 5–8.

Luker K.A. (1985) Evaluating health visiting practice. In Luker K.A. & Orr J. (eds.) *Health Visiting,* 1st edn. Oxford, Blackwell Scientific Publications.

Luker K.A. & Caress A-L. (1989) Rethinking patient education. *Journal of Advanced Nursing* **14**, 711–18.

McFarlane J.K. (1977) Developing a theory of nursing the relation of theory to practice Education and research. *Journal of Advanced Nursing* **2**(3), 261–70.

MacIntyre S. (1976) Who wants babies. The social construction of instincts. In Baker A. & Allen T. (eds.) *Sexual Division in Society: Process and Change.* Tavistock, London.

MacIntyre S. (1977) *Single and Pregnant.* Croom Helm, London.

MacIver R.M. & Page C.H. (1961) *Society.* Macmillan, London.

Magee B. (1973) *Popper.* Fontana/Collins, Glasgow.

Marans R.W. (1976) Perceived quality of residential environments; some methodological issues. In Craik K. & Zube E. (eds.) *Perceiving Environmental Quality Research and Applications.* Plenum Press, New York.

Marris T. (1971) *The Work of the Health Visitors in London.* Research Report No. 12, Greater London Department of Planning and Transportation, London.

Mayers M. (1972) Programme evaluation in community health a search for assessment criteria. *Nursing Outlook* **20**(5), 323-6.

Mayo M. (1977) *Women in the Community.* Routledge & Kegan Paul, London.

McCall J. (1988) Evaluating Quality. *Senior Nurse* **8**(5), 8-9.

Midwinter E. (1973) *Patterns of Community Education.* Ward Lock Publications, London.

Milio N. (1976) A framework for prevention: changing health damaging to health generating patterns. *American Journal of Public Health* **66**(5), 435-9.

Milio N. (1986) *Promoting health through public policy*, 2nd edn. Ottawa Canadian Public Health Association.

Millar B. (1989a) Making sense of resource management. *Nursing Times* **85** (11); 26-32.

Millar B. & Sheldon T. (1989b) Caring for people a framework for the future. *Health Service Journal* **99** (5178); 1422-5.

Miller A. (1985) Nurse-patient dependency is it iatrogenic? *Journal of Advanced Nursing* **10**; 63-9.

Moos R.H. (1976) *The Human Context; Environmental Determinants of Behaviour.* John Wiley, New York.

Moran G. (1991) Fourth time around: NHS re-organisation and public health. In *Health through public policy*, (Ed. by P. Draper), Green Print, London.

Morrison D. & Betts A. (1990) The Wessex computer assisted learning project. *Information Technology in Nursing* **2**(2); 19-22.

Murphy J.F. (1971) *Theoretical Issues in Professional Nursing.* Appleton Century Crofts, New York.

Mussallem H.K. (1988) Prevention and patterns of disease. In *Recent advances in nursing, prevention and nursing* (Ed. by R. Willis & J. Linwood), Churchill Livingstone, Edinburgh.

Newby H. & Bell C. (1971) *Community Studies.* Allen and Unwin, London.

NHS Management Executive (1991) *ADHA Project Paper: Moving Forward, Needs, Services and Contracts.* NHS Management Executive, Richmond House, London.

Oakley A. (1974) *The Sociology of Housework.* Martin Robertson, Oxford.

Oakley A. (1980) *Women Confined: Towards a Sociology of Childbirth.* Martin Robertson, Oxford.

Open University (1985a) *Medical Knowledge: Doubt and Certainty*, Book 2 of U205 Health and Disease, Open University Press, Milton Keynes.

Open University (1985b) *Experiencing and Explaining Disease*, Book 6 of U205 Health and Disease, Open University Press, Milton Keynes.

Orem D. (1971) *Nursing Concepts of Practice.* McGraw Hill, New York.

Orr J. (1980) *Health Visiting in Focus.* Royal College of Nursing, London.

Orr J. (1982) Feminism and health visiting. Health Visitor **54**(4), 156-7.

Orr J. (1983) Is health visiting meeting today's needs? *Health Visitor* **56**(6), 200-3.

Orr J. (1985) The community dimension. In *Health Visiting* 1st edn (Ed. by K.A. Luker & J. Orr). Blackwell Scientific Publications, Oxford.

Orr J. (1987) *Women's health in the community.* J. Wiley, Chichester.

Orr J. (1988) Women's health: A nursing perspective. In *Political Issues in Nursing; Past, Present and Future*, Vol. 3 (Ed. by R. White). J. Wiley, Chichester.

Pahl R.E. (1970) *Patterns of Urban Life.* Longman, London.

Phaneuf M.C. (1976) *The Nursing Audit: Self-regulation in Nursing Practice* (2nd edn). Appléton Century Crofts, New York.

Plant R. (1978) Community: concept, conception and ideology. *Politics and Society* **8**(1), 79-107.

Plant R., Lesser H. & Taylor-Gooby P. (1980) *Political Philosophy and Social Welfare.* Routledge & Kegan Paul, London.

Pinker R. (1982) An alternative view: appendix B. In *Social Workers: Their Role and Tasks*, National Institute for Social Work. Bedford Press, London.

Poulton K. (1977) *Evaluation of Community Nursing Services of Wandsworth and East Merton Teaching District.* (Unpublished research report.)

Reading: County Council and Area Health Authorities of Berkshire and Hampshire (1979) *Report of the Inquiry into the death of Lester Chapman.*

Report of the Committee on Local Authority and Allied Personal Social Services (1968) (Seebohm Report) CMND 3703 HMSO, London.

Reid D. & Holland W. (1978) Measurement in Health Care Studies. In Holland W. & Karhausen L. (eds.) *Health Care and Epidemiology.* Henry Kimpton, London.

Reilly D. (1975) Why a conceptual framework? *Nursing Outlook* **23**(8), 566-9.

Riecken H.W. (1952) *The Volunteer Work Camp: A Psychological Evaluation.* Addison Wesley Press, Cambridge, Massachusetts.

Riehl S. & Roy C. (1980) *Conceptual Models for Nursing Practice* (2nd edn). Appleton Century Crofts, New York.

Rimmer L. (1983) The economics of work and caring. In Finch J. & Groves D. (eds.) *A Labour of Love Women, Work and Caring.* Routledge & Kegan Paul, London.

Roberts D.E. (1962) How effective is public health nursing? *American Journal of Public Health* **52**(7), 1077-83.

Robinson J. (1982) *An Evaluation of Health Visiting.* Council for the Education and Training of Health Visitors, London.

Robinson J. (1985) Health visiting and health. In *Political Issues in Nursing Past, Present and Future* (Ed. by R. White). John Wiley & Sons, Chichester.

Robinson K.S.M. (1986) The Social Construction of Health Visiting. Unpublished PhD Thesis, South Bank Polytechnic.

Robinson K. & Vaughan B. (eds) (1992) *Knowledge for Nursing.* Heinemann, Oxford.

Rosenstock I. (1966) *Why People Use Health Services.* Health Services Research Study Project. Public Health Services, New York.

Rosenthal H. (1983) Neighbourhood Health Projects. Some new approaches to health and community work in parts of the United Kingdom. *Community Development Journal* 18(2), 120-31.

Rossiter C. & Wicks M. (1982) *Crisis or Challenge? Family Care, Elderly People and Social Policy.* Study Commission on the Family, London.

Roy C. (1976) *Introduction to Nursing: an Adaptation Model.* Prentice Hall, New York.

Roy S. (1990) Nursing in the community, Sheila Roy, Director of Nursing, NW Thames RHA.

Ryle G. (1963) *The Concept of Mind.* Penguin, Harmondsworth.

Sachs H. (1990) A brave attempt: teamwork between health visitors and social workers on an inner city estate. *King's Fund Centre,* London.

Saddington N. (1984) Putting Korner into practice. *Nursing Times* 80(22); 53-5.

Schroyer T. (1971) The critical theory of later capitalism. In Fisher G. (ed.) *The Revival of American Socialism.* Oxford University Press, New York.

Schuck P.H. (1977) Public interest groups and the policy process. *Public Administration Review* (March/April), 132-40.

Schulberg H.C. & Baker F.G. (1968) Programme Evaluation Models and the Implementation of Research Findings. *American Journal of Public Health* 58(7) 1255-98.

Schutz A. (1964) The stranger: an essay in social psychology. In Brodesen A. (ed.) *Studies in Social Theory* (collected papers II), 91-105. Martinus Nijhoff, The Hague.

Schwirian P.M., Malone J.A., Stone V.S., Nunley B. & Francisco T. (1989) Computers in nursing practice a comparison of attitudes of nurses and nursing students. *Computers in Nursing* 7(4); 168-77.

Shapiro S. (1977) Measuring the effectiveness of prevention II. *Milbank Memorial Fund Quarterly Health and Society* (Spring), 291-308.

Sharp R. & Green A. (1975) *Education and Social Control.* Routledge & Kegan Paul, London.

Sharrock W.W. (1974) On owning knowledge. In Turner R. (ed.) *Ethnomethodology.* Penguin, Harmondsworth.

Shibutani T. (1955) Reference groups as perspectives. In Manis I.G. & Meltzer B.N. (eds.) *Symbolic Interaction.* Allyn & Bacon, Boston.

Smith A. & Jacobson B. (Eds.) (1988) *The nation's health: a strategy for the 1990s.* Oxford University Press, Oxford.

Society of Family Practitioner Committees (1989) The 1990 General Medical Practitioners Contract *NAHA Briefing* n20.

Speakman J. (1984) Measuring the immeasurable. *Nursing Times* 80(22); 56-8.

Spencer B., Gray J., Dunham M. & Jones V. (1982) *An Evaluation of the Manchester Well Woman Clinic.* Unpublished Report.

Spender D. (1980) *Man Made Language.* Routledge & Kegan Paul, London.

Startsman T.S. & Robinson R.E. (1972) Attitudes of medical and paramedical personnel toward computers. *Computers and Biomedical Research* 5;

218-27.

Stimpson G.V. (1974) Obeying Doctor's orders: A view from the other side. *Social Science and Medicine,* **18**, 97-104.

Stronge J.H. & Brodt A. (1985) Assessment of nurses attitudes toward computerisation. *Computers in Nursing* **3**; 154-8.

Stuart A. & Sundeen M. (1979) *Principles and Practice of Psychiatric Nursing.* C.V. Mosby, St. Louis.

Suchman E.A. (1967) *Evaluation Research.* Russell Sage Foundation, New York.

Sultana, N. (1990) Nurses attitudes toward computerisation in clinical practice. *Journal of Advanced Nursing* **15**; 696-702.

Thayer R. (1973) Measuring need in the social services. *Social and Economic Administration* (7 May) 91-105.

Thies J.B. (1975) Hospital personnel and computer based systems a study of attitudes and perceptions. *Hospital Administration* **20**; 17-26.

Thomas B. (1985) A survey study of computers in nursing. *Computers in Nursing* **3**; 173 9.

Thomas B. (1989) Development of an instrument to assess attitudes toward computing in nursing. *Computers in Nursing* **6**(3); 122-7.

Thunhurst C. (1985) The analysis of small area statistics and planning for health. *The Statistician,* **34**, 187-200.

Titmuss R.M. (1974) *Social Policy.* Allen & Unwin, London.

Tonnies F. (1955 - first published in 1887) *Community and Association.* Routledge & Kegan Paul, London.

Tucker W.H. (1979) The nature of a community. In Fromer M.J. (ed.) *Community health care and the nursing process.* C.V. Mosby, St. Louis.

United Kingdom Central Council (1990) *Post Registration Education and Practice Project* (PREPP). UKCC, London.

United Kingdom Central Council (1991) *Report on Proposals for the Future of Community Education and Practice,* UKCC, London.

United States Department of Health, Education and Welfare (1969) *Towards a social report.* Washington D.C., United States of America.

Urban Programme Circular No. 1 (1968) Home Office. HMSO, London.

Wall T.D. (1987) New technology and job design. *Psychology at Work* (Ed. by P.B. Warr). Penguin, Harmondsworth.

Weaver BN.R. (1977) Conceptual basis for nursing intervention with human systems: communities and societies. In Hall J.E. & Weaver B.R. (eds.), *Distributive Nursing Practice: a Systems Approach to Community Health.* J.B. Lippincott Co., Philadelphia.

Weed L.L. (1969) *Medical Records, Medical Education and Patient Care.* Press of Case Western Reserve University, Ohio.

Weiner R. (1975) *The Rape and Plunder of the Shankhill.* Notarms Press, Belfast

Wellman B. & Leighton B. (1979) Networks, neighbourhoods and communities. *Urban Affairs Quarterly* **14**(3), 363-900.

Whitehouse C.R. (1981) Preparing to introduce a computer into a health centre. *British Medical Journal* **283**; 197-210.

Wiedenback A. & Fall P. (1978) *Communication Key to Effective Nursing.*

Triesias Press, New York.

Wilding P. (1982) *Professional Power and Social Welfare*. Routledge & Kegan Paul, London.

Wise D. (1991) The smart set who are playing their cards right. *The Guardian* (44905) 30.1.91.

Wiseman J. (1979) Activities and priorities of health visitors 1–2, *Nursing Times Occasional Paper* **75**, 24–5.

Wiseman J. (1990) Get smart. *British Journal of Health Care Computing* **7**(5); 21–3.

World Health Organisation (1946) Constitution. WHO, Geneva.

World Health Organisation (1974) *Community Health Nursing*. Report of a WHO Expert Committee, Technical Report Series 556, WHO, Geneva.

World Health Organisation (1978) *Primary Health Care*. A joint report by the Director-General of the World Health Organisation and the Executive Director of United Nations Children's fund. World Health Organisation, Geneva.

World Health Organisation (1979) *Regional Workshop on Nursing and Midwifery Personnel in Primary Health Care*. World Health Organisation, Manila.

World Health Organisation (1981) *Global Strategy for Health for All by the Year 2000*. WHO, Geneva.

World Health Organisation (1984) *Having a Baby in Europe*. World Health Organisation, Geneva.

World Health Organisation (1985a) *Women's Health and Development*, a report by the Director General WHO, Geneva.

World Health Organisation (1986) *Nursing and the 38 Targets of Health for All – A discussion paper*. Nursing Unit, WHO/Euro, Copenhagen.

World Health Organisation (1986) Health and Welfare Canada, Canadian Public Health Association *Ottawa Charter for Health Promotion* WHO/Euro, Copenhagen.

World Health Organisation (1988) *Appropriate information systems for primary health care*. WHO, Geneva.

Wright P. & Treacher A. (1982) *The Problem of Medical Knowledge*. University of Edinburgh Press, Edinburgh.

Zielstorff R.D. (1984) Why aren't there more significant automated nursing information systems? *Journal of Nursing Administration* **14**(1); 7–10.

Zimmer M.J. (1974) Guidelines for development of outcome criteria. *Nursing Clinics of North America* **9**(2), 317–21.

Zola I.K. (1972) Medicine as an Institution of Social Control. *Sociological Review* **20**(4), 487–504.

Index

PROPERTY OF MEDICAL LIBRARY
WEST MIDDLESEX HOSPITAL,
ISLEWORTH.